What I've
Learned *from*
You

What I've Learned from You

The Lessons of Life Taught to a Doctor by His Patients

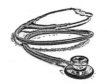

SCOTT A. KELLY, M.D.

FOREWORD BY BERNIE SIEGEL, M.D.

ART HEALS MEDIA

ISBN 978-0-9912743-2-1

Book design by Karen Minster

Printed in the United States of America

First Printing, 2015

Art Heals Media, Inc.
553 Peachtree Battle Avenue
Atlanta, Ga. 30305

For Caelyn and Elizabeth, my angels on earth.

And for Deborah, forever.

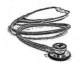

Knowledge of our own mortality
is the greatest gift God ever gives us.

—Anna Quindlen

CONTENTS

FOREWORD

Bernie Siegel, M.D.

AUTHOR OF *LOVE, MEDICINE, & MIRACLES*
AND *THE ART OF HEALING*

SCOTT'S BOOK SAYS IT ALL. I LEARNED THESE LESSONS MANY years ago. We receive medical information but not an education in medical school. We are trained to treat the result and not the cause. Physicians need to be taught how to care for themselves and their patients. The practice of medicine needs to be about people.

When I ask medical students to draw themselves working as a doctor they draw medical equipment, themselves, a desk, and a diploma on the wall. It is a rare student who is seen with a patient and treating that patient like a human being. A good physician helps patients find their self-esteem and love themselves. Physicians should help patients see how their lives can contribute to the onset of illness without guilt becoming an issue. Physicians should teach patients to survive.

Hope is not a statistical issue. It is about faith and human potential. Patient and doctors should be a team who communicate with one another. Survivors take responsibility for their life and work with their physicians as a team. They coach each other. Death is not a failure.

In Thornton Wilder's one-act play *The Angel That Troubled the Waters*, the angel refuses to allow the physician to be healed. The angel says "Without your wound where would your power be? . . . In love's service, only wounded soldiers can serve." I believe every doctor should be a hospital patient for a week. It would be a gift to both patients and physicians.

What I've Learned from You can teach us all to learn from one another.

A NOTE FROM THE AUTHOR

THE STORIES YOU WILL READ IN *WHAT I'VE LEARNED FROM YOU* are based on real patients. You might ask, "What about the doctor-patient relationship?"

Excellent question.

How do I protect patient confidentiality but retain the essence of truth? I came up with the following with the help of friends, writers, lawyers, and the advice of a select group of my patients. The names have been changed, and some of the situations have been altered—occasionally also the genders—in order to protect patient confidentiality and to retain trust. The time line remains relatively intact.

After all, I plan on practicing medicine for a long time, and I don't want my patients worried that they'll be a chapter in my next book. The physician-patient relationship has enough challenges looming on the horizon. It needs to be nourished, respected, and protected.

Information not disclosed to me during the physician-patient relationship was obtained through research. I reviewed obituaries, relied on the memory of my colleagues, and interviewed family members. I did this to best represent my patients.

I reserve literary right to delete, subtract, or add information to make the story more intriguing for the reader. I did my best to retain the truth and honor the physician-patient relationship. I feel strongly that these stories need to be told, because without sharing them they, like all of us, will perish.

And I believe they deserve to live.

INTRODUCTION

LATE ONE NIGHT, WHILE SORTING THROUGH BOXES IN THE attic, I found an old journal. I brushed the back of my hand across the weathered leather. The hand-stitching was unraveled, the binder broken, the leather faded and splintered. I crouched down on the plywood floor and sat among the scattered cardboard boxes as my eyes slowly adjusted to the dimness of the light.

I smiled as I leafed through the pages. At the top of the first page, I had once written the words *What I've Learned from You*. As I read the stories, a wave of nostalgia overcame me… a vestige of a very different time of my life.

I closed my eyes, and in the theater of my mind I saw the first time I had written in my journal. It was the fall of 1994, and I had entered my third year of medical school. The once leafy trees were barren, and the grass was littered with gold and rust remnants. On my desk sat a pile of class notes and textbooks. Examinations were approaching, and I was overwhelmed.

I had leaned back in my chair and stared at the ceiling. For the first time in my life, I had wondered if becoming a doctor was the right decision. A feeling had consumed me—the feeling that something in my life, a part of me, was missing—an unmistakable but palpable void.

I'd looked out my office window and seen a young boy playing in his front yard. He threw a red rubber ball into the air, then ran beneath it with outstretched arms. As he caught it and the ball thumped against his chest, he laughed and smiled. In that moment, I'd realized what I was missing . . . I'd lost my smile. I'd wondered what happened to the little boy inside me.

I had walked over to my bookshelf and picked up my journal and begun writing. It was my way of dealing with pain. Writing clarified my thoughts. It helped me to see the world more clearly and provided companionship in times of loneliness.

In those days, I didn't feel like I had the time to invest in personal growth, so I had reached out to those around me. My patients, the ones who were hurting the most, were the first to embrace me. My patients had become my teachers. Even in their darkest moments, they'd opened their hearts and exposed their wounds. I had listened and paid attention, and I had written in my journal what I had learned.

After finding my old journal in 2006, I began rewriting the stories to share with my children. Maybe they could learn from them too. I hoped my patients' experiences would help ease their transition through life and serve as a reference when the world was unkind. Just in case I wasn't there to teach them.

But the challenge was daunting. The encounters had occurred throughout many different times in my life—medical school, residency, and the first years of private practice. How could I unify a collection of stories? Over the years, I wrote out the stories in bits and pieces in the hope of finding a common thread. And in a beautiful way, the thread appeared. The stories wrote themselves.

Now I share them with you, so that we can all learn from the wisdom and experiences of these remarkable individuals. Following each story, I added a reflection on the experience. An observation from a life lived in medicine. Sometimes my perception of the lesson had changed. I'll share that with you too. Each and every day, I am still learning. I remain a work in progress.

What I've Learned from You is the story of human experience. It is the story of love and pain and healing and sickness and birth and death and all of the beautiful things in between. It is a front-row seat into the window of the human condition.

The answers to life's questions are all around us. They lie within each of us. We need to open our hearts and pay attention to one another. I know this to be true.

My patients taught me so.

PREFACE

IT'S THE FIRST DAY OF MEDICAL SCHOOL IN OUR FIRST YEAR at the Medical College of Georgia in August of 1992. We file into the air-conditioned auditorium. Outside, the humidity is intense, the sun relentless. We sit perched on the edge of our seats; adrenaline pumps through our bodies, much as it does in athletes before they step onto the field.

Through the side door, our head anatomy professor, Dr. Gene Colborn, walks in: silver hair, short stature, rounding shoulders, and a commanding presence. His assistants follow him—the room silences. He walks to the front and stands behind a silver table with a white body bag lying on it. He approaches the microphone and brings it close to his mouth.

"Ladies and gentlemen, welcome to medical school."

He pauses just long enough to take in the sea of students in front of him.

"In front of me lies a woman who died in our university hospital last night." He looks up at us. "She has graciously donated her body to science, so that you can learn from her... We expect you to treat your cadavers with respect—as you would a family member."

I sit back from the edge of my seat and take a deep breath. I realize there is no way I could have prepared for what I am about to go through.

What I've
Learned
from
You

Unraveling the Connection between Mind and Body

Body and soul cannot be separated for purposes
of treatment, for they are one and indivisible.

— C. Jeff Miller

It's a warm summer Friday evening in 1992, and Dr. Thomas
Weidman stands at the top of a cadaver's table with a human
brain in his hand. Our anatomy exams for our first year of medical school begin on Monday. Dr. Weidman chooses to spend the
evening with his students rather than at home. As an assistant
anatomy professor, he helps write the exams and knows this one is
particularly tough. He wants us to be prepared.

Staring at him, I can't help but notice his appearance. He
doesn't look much like a professor. He's short, bald, shaped like a
pear, and waddles when he walks. Arthritis has settled into his
hips and knees, but his physical appearance is deceiving. He's as
sharp as a tack, and his wit is unparalleled. He is a gifted teacher
who can bring home a point like no one else.

Students gather around him and take notes at a feverish
pace. He pulls a silver instrument from a tub, and the smell of

formaldehyde fills our noses. He points the instrument at the base of the brain. "This is the brain stem. Tell me exactly what it does."

"It controls blood pressure, breathing, and heart rate," a student says.

"Good, those are the important ones." He points to the cerebellum at the back of the base of the brain. "And this."

"The cerebellum. It controls coordination and balance."

He nods.

He points to the front of the brain. No one responds. "Ever gone to a party and ended up getting naked and jumping into the pool?"

All the medical students stiffen up, and no one raises their hand. "Well, if you did . . ." He points to the front of the brain, to the frontal cortex. "This would be the part of the brain that was uninhibited from the cocktails you drank at the party."

Everyone chuckles and looks at one another. He never cracks a smile.

"How about this one, then? Same part of the brain, but it also controls something else." No one responds. "Ever lost someone you love, and you get that feeling—in the pit of your stomach?" People nod their heads gently so others won't see. But there are so many heads moving that everyone can't help but notice a general sense of agreement. "Well, this is also the place of feelings, or emotions. This is where it begins." His voice drops to a whisper. "Long before it takes that permanent place in your heart."

He clears his throat gently, and I see the corners of his eyes well with tears. He quickly regains his composure and continues on.

Fall of 1994

Third Year of Medical School

BERNIE SAT BACK IN HIS CHAIR AND STARED OUT OF THE hospital room window. It was a pale, gray October day, and he watched the trees gently sway back and forth. Bernie's mood was reflective. He was distant, guarded, and introspective.

"How are you feeling?" I asked.

Silence filled the room. He waited for what seemed like an eternity before he acknowledged my presence.

"Doctor, do you believe in the mind-body connection?" His eyes shifted from the window to his interlocked fingers resting in his lap.

"No," I responded. An instinctive response without thought.

His face was void of expression. His eyes rolled and then seemed to sink deeper within their sockets. Each rare movement of his long, lanky arms was slow and deliberate. His dark-brown hair spilled into his eyes and tangled with his beard.

Although his body lumbered along in slow motion, I sensed the racing of his thoughts. From the moment he placed his first foot on the floor to the moment the nurse quietly turned his reading light off, Bernie's mind never took a break. Little by little his thoughts consumed him.

Bernie had never planned on being in the hospital. On a crisp fall night, on his way to a coffee shop, he'd stumbled upon two strangers in an altercation. One of the men pulled out a gun and fired. A stray bullet found its way into Bernie's abdomen. Both men ran.

A trauma surgeon had met him at the door of the Emergency Room, and through five grueling hours of surgery, he carefully put Bernie's torn blood vessels back together. He'd removed his spleen and repaired his stomach. Bernie received five pints of blood and spent ten days in intensive care. Rehabilitation had taken another two weeks.

I'd taken over his care as a medical student on a general surgery rotation. The hours were long, and as soon as one patient was stabilized, two more were waiting. We students had felt like we were drowning, and just as we were about to suffocate, we'd be given one last breath of air. The sea had quickly pulled us back beneath the surface.

I'd tried each morning to engage Bernie in conversation, but my attempts were often ignored. I'd respected his need for distance and privacy. He'd seemed to want to be alone in his thoughts. I had understood. I often feel the same.

Bernie's words continued to find their place at the forefront of my thoughts—in the drive home from the hospital that night, in the middle of conversation with others, and sometimes in the loneliness of night when I couldn't sleep. "Doctor, do you believe in the mind-body connection?" His words quietly floated through my mind.

Early one Tuesday morning, just after sunrise, I eased into his room. The sun's orange glare cast a thin ray of light as it shone through the curtains. I checked his vital signs and tried not to wake him. His body slowly stirred in bed.

"Go back to sleep," I said. "I'm sorry; it's early."

"It's all right. I had a hard time sleeping anyway," he said. He rolled over and reached for his bedside table. His long, thin fingers fumbled with his glasses. He seemed like a new person: his mannerisms, his voice, and the way he sprang up to sit in his bed. It was evident he had something to say. His distant and cold demeanor had evaporated. His mind was lucid and sharp.

"Do you remember when I asked you about the mind-body connection?"

"I do." My head tilted toward the ground.

"Well, explain something to me. Let's say I say something to you and you become embarrassed. You blush, right?" he said. "What happened?"

"Well, your mind interprets an external stimulus and your body responds."

"Exactly," he said. "And let's say you are at the theater, and a scene in a movie scares you. Do you cringe in your seat?"

"I do."

"So what happened there?"

"Same thing. Your mind interprets an external stimulus, and your body responds."

"You are beginning to understand." His smile broadened. He was now fully awake.

"Can you help me up, over there to that chair?" he asked.

I placed my arm out for support. He grabbed on, and then I placed my hand over his arm and held him firmly.

He walked over to the window and looked down across the buildings of the hospital's campus. The sun had worked its way toward the top of the tall pine trees and cast a shadow across the lawn. The first signs of life emerged around campus: An athletic team ran in two lines—side by side—down the sidewalk, a few scattered students headed out to study, drivers headed off on their way to work as their cars' white headlights cut through the last bit of fog. His eyes scanned the scene beneath him.

"I need my doctor to understand that there is a mind-body connection. My injury affects me just as much emotionally as it does physically. They go hand in hand. At times I'm angry and depressed. I'm lacking trust right now in others. Sometimes I feel lucky to be alive. Sometimes I wish I had died. The physical pain is not the half of it. The emotional pain is often worse. I can wrap my mind around the physical pain." He turned his head toward me. He looked winded.

"I understand," I said, as I looked him directly in the eyes. "And…I'm sorry I said what I did."

I helped him to a seat by the window. He leaned forward and rested his elbow on the windowsill. "When I leave here, I will work on regaining trust in others. My life changed in a matter of moments from two people I had never met. When I got shot, instead of helping me, they ran. I still have to deal with that."

His mood was somber. I felt his pain as if it were my own.

"Why do you believe that doctors have a hard time believing in things they can't explain? If it's not supported by the medical literature, it doesn't exist?"

"Bernie, I don't know… maybe it's the way we're taught," I said.

"These theories—are they written by people who take care of patients or by scientists?"

"Mostly scientists."

"Figures. They would never say that if they were sitting where I am—take this for what it's worth. Once you become a patient, everything you thought was important in life … well, it doesn't really matter. It's the heart that matters," he said. "Be a doctor with heart."

I looked over his shoulder out the window of his room. The sun had risen, and a new day was upon us. And from that moment on, I never thought about the theory of the mind-body connection the same way again.

We are just scratching the surface of understanding the science behind the relationship between emotions and the human condition. We still have much to learn. Bernie taught me that the mind-body connection exists. How do I know for sure?

My mind believes it, and my heart responds.

∽

THE DAY BERNIE LEFT THE HOSPITAL HE REACHED HIS HAND out to me. "Always remember what I told you," he said. I assured him I would. He pointed to his heart. "And carry it in here, wherever you may go."

Bernie taught me the importance of understanding the intimate connection between the mind and body. How an illness manifests into the arena of our lives. How the issues of acceptance and trust and hope and faith all play a part. How illness can drain our self-esteem and spill over into our relationships with our significant others, friends, children, and colleagues.

It was a lesson my dear professor of anatomy, Dr. Thomas Weidman, had tried to teach us too.

While researching this book, I discovered that Dr. Thomas Weidman had passed away in 2002. His colleague and friend, Dr. Gene L. Colborn, wrote an obituary. It began: "Even before the break of daylight and into the evening hours, he was there for his students. We, his friends and colleagues, are grateful that he was there for us too."

I thought of that Friday evening with Dr. Weidman in the cadaver lab. I remember him being there for his students even though he wasn't required to be. I recall the way he used humor to bring his point across. In his own subtle way, he taught us about the intimate connection between the mind and the body. He wanted us to recognize the connection between thoughts, feelings, emotions, and illness.

As a professor, he knew the anatomy of the human body better than anyone, yet he was silently suffering from prostate cancer. In his private life, alone with his wife and family, he knew the side of being a patient too.

Dr. Colburn ended his obituary with "Tom left his life with gentle acceptance, still possessing his delightful sense of humor and, understandably, with no misgivings for what was to come. We will not, cannot, forget what he shared with us."

Nor will I.

Finding Strength

The worst thing, of course—
and you're never quite prepared for it—
is when the patient dies during the operation.
You die a little every time that happens.

— MICHAEL DEBAKEY, M.D., HEART SURGEON

It's July of 1991, my senior year of college at Emory University in Atlanta, Georgia. It's time for us students to choose our classes for the fall semester. We stare at the long lists of classes while in a hot, sweaty gym. We fan our faces with class schedules to keep cool. As my eyes scan the list of classes, one title keeps catching my eye. Fine, I figure, if I'm going to be a doctor, I need to learn about death and dying. The last class I pencil in is a religion class entitled Death and Dying.

The first day of class we sit in wooden chairs in a circle. My professor enters the room. He is a tall man with silver, thinning hair. He wears a tweed sport coat with sleeves that stop well short of his wrists. The legs of his pants don't quite meet his ankles. He sits right in the middle of the circle, with his chair backward. He scans the room, making sure he looks each of us in the eyes.

"Students… my friends," he begins. "You signed up for a class called Death and Dying. And, yes, it is true we will be talking about death and dying. But my greatest goal of this course is for you to understand that by learning about death you can learn to live. You can live purposefully and with conviction— and not have to be confronted by an illness or death in order to allow yourself to live life in a meaningful manner."

A part of me was relieved. A part of me wondered if I had signed up for the wrong class.

Fall of 1994

Third Year of Medical School

IT WAS JUST AFTER TWO THIRTY IN THE MORNING WHEN Chris lifted his head out of the toilet for the third time that night. He'd awakened with a headache, but his head now felt like it was going to explode. His wife came into the bathroom and knelt beside him.

"Will you take me to the emergency room?" he asked.

The moment his wife, Anna, heard those words, she knew their life would never be the same. Chris rarely complained and never showed pain. As a college football player, he'd once played an entire game with a broken bone in his foot and a torn rotator cuff. It had been the last game of the season. "The body will heal if you let it," he would say. It had. This time was different. He knew something was terribly wrong and he needed help. This time the body couldn't heal itself.

That night, an astute emergency room physician ordered a CT scan of his brain. It lit up a large, suspicious mass. An MRI confirmed a tumor a few millimeters short of the size of a baseball.

The moment the physician told Chris, his body went numb. He choked up and had trouble finding words. His wife broke down in tears. Chris promised her that he would find a way to make it. For his entire life, he'd always been in control. Secretly, now, he felt his control silently slipping.

"I'll fight. No matter what, I'll fight."

Chris fought with every ounce of strength within his soul. By the time I met him he had undergone three brain surgeries, plus chemotherapy and radiation. He was undergoing rehabilitation to regain his strength. The neurosurgeon had given him six months to live, and he was well into his fifth month. He continued fighting.

In my third week of taking care of Chris, the Atlanta Braves were making an October run at the World Series. The town buzzed with excitement. The fans lined Peachtree Street, going from tavern to tavern. People leaned out of their cars' sunroofs and beeped their horns in celebration.

"Are you on call tonight?" Chris asked.

"I am."

"Well, if you get bored, you're welcome to come down and watch the game with me."

"Thanks. If I can get away for a few minutes, I just might do that," I said.

That evening, just before game time, I knocked on his door. "Do you still want some company?"

"Sure—pull up a seat."

During the second inning, our conversation turned toward life, love, and dying. By the fourth inning, we had switched off the television.

"I am so sorry this happened to you," I said. The words just rolled off my tongue without a thought.

"Yeah, me too," he said. "Me too." He was so tall that his feet hung off the end of the bed. He sat upright with his shoulders resting against the wall. "I remember that night in the emergency room so well. It's one of those moments you never forget. When they wheeled me from the room where they did the CAT scan, I could see my pictures. Even I could see the mass in my brain. But even though I saw it, I didn't want to believe it was mine. The interesting thing about all this—the dying—it's not exactly like what you would think. It just doesn't seem real. Forty years on this earth is not enough. We all know we're going to die, but we never really believe it," he said.

We sat in silence for a moment.

"I try not to think about it too much, but sometimes I just can't help myself. I miss my wife and my daughter, and I'm not even gone yet," he said.

I sat back and listened to him. I was aware of the fact that it could just as easily be me sitting in that bed, with the scar across my head, wishing for a miracle.

"I would give anything, and I do mean anything, for just more time—just so I could be with my wife and daughter a little longer."

He sank into his bed and thought for a moment. "You know, I've never taken my daughter to Disney World. I never got to see her perform at her ballet recital. I'd love to hear her play violin—she'll be starting lessons soon," he said. "I want to see her get married. I want to meet my grandchildren."

As I expected, Chris kept fighting. With each new challenge he came out swinging and somehow found a way to make it through.

After rehabilitation made him more functional, he was discharged from the hospital. Two months later, as I completed a consultation in the hospital, a code was called. A patient had gone into cardiac arrest, and I went to see if I could be of assistance. As I turned the corner I saw Chris's wife standing outside the door, tears streaming down her face, and I realized that it was Chris in cardiac arrest. I never knew he was back in the hospital.

I looked at her for a moment, and then I rushed into the room and placed my arm on his shoulder.

"Chris!" I screamed. "Chris!"

He didn't respond. I then squeezed his shoulder. His head fell and rested against my forearm. That was the last response from Chris. After many rounds of shocks with paddles that lifted his lifeless body off the bed, and drugs pumped through his body to restart his heart, he never responded. I placed his head against the pillow.

Despite our best efforts, Chris didn't make it. He left behind a beautiful wife and a young daughter. And I silently prayed that he had moved on to a better place.

I went to a small, empty room, laid my face within my hands, and cried. I had let my guard down and was hurt. It had affected me. Chris was the first person I'd watched die right in front of me. I'd watched as he took his last breath, and I'd watched as his body went limp and cold. And I felt like a failure for not being able to save him. I felt angry and helpless and sad and alone.

Nothing had prepared me for the pain.

∽

RECENTLY, A FRIEND ASKED ME HOW I SEPARATE MY LIFE AS A physician from my home life. How do I leave my work at the office? The first person to enter my mind was Chris. His death has forever impacted me. The picture of him lying there in bed after he passed is forever imprinted on my mind.

The truth is I do a terrible job of separating my work and life. A part of me wishes I could leave everything at the office, but I've accepted that I can't. At times I'm not so sure that I should, and I've come to terms with my own limitations.

Chris reminded me to embrace life. To do those things in life that I've always wanted to do. As I age, and the list of things I want to do in life grows, I look around me. I see people in my peer group diagnosed with fatal illnesses, and the brevity of life settles in.

Yet, somehow, I still seem to be able to find a distance between a patient's mortality and my own. A self-induced denial mechanism that helps me cope with the inevitable. But when I sit here and think of Chris and the day I tried to bring him back to life and couldn't, my mind so easily slips back into that moment.

I look at my wife and my daughters and know exactly how he felt.

Light at the
End of the Tunnel

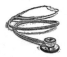

Character consists of what you do
on the third and fourth tries.

—James Michener

It's just after eight o'clock on the first morning of exams in our first year of medical school in 1992. The last three months of our lives were spent learning about the anatomy of the human body. Now it's time to show what we remember.

We enter the anatomy lab in single file. The room is filled with cadavers lying on rows of stainless-steel tables. A white tag sits on each anatomical part we are to name. We have thirty seconds at each table and then a bell rings. Time to move on to the next table. If the answer doesn't jump into your mind, you are not allowed to return.

A medical student in front of me is frustrated. I can tell by his breathing and the way he shakes his head. The bell rings. When we approach the sixth table, he takes his clipboard and steps back. He drops his clipboard into a big metal sink, and the clamoring of metal on metal ensues. I see his paper is blank.

He hangs his white coat on a hook and walks out the door. He has decided at that moment that he no longer wants to become a doctor.

I never saw him again, but occasionally the thought of him crosses my mind—in those moments when I feel great personal satisfaction with the privilege of being a physician. I'm curious if he regrets his decision. But most of all, I wonder about how many people he could have helped if he'd decided to stay.

Spring of 1995

Third Year of Medical School

WALTER SPENT THE GREATER YEARS OF HIS LIFE MASTER-ing the art of surgery. But one day, in the middle of a case, a tremor overtook his hand. The tremor began gradually over a few weeks, but he'd always been able to suppress it. This time he couldn't. He almost dropped the scalpel. At that moment, he knew his days of operating were over.

"I need you to call my partner and tell him to come to the operating room," he calmly told the nurse.

His partner finished the case while Walter watched. That was the last day he operated. That afternoon he called his friend, a neurologist. "I need you to see me ... I have a problem."

The next morning he found himself in his friend's office and they went through his history. At sixty-four his body was beginning to fail him. His feet shuffled when he walked. At times he almost fell. He reached out for guardrails and furniture to provide support. He no longer drank his evening Scotch, as he needed all the stability his body could muster. He needed help getting out of his car. He had trouble holding a toothbrush and combing his silver hair.

The doctor made Walter walk across the room. He asked him to hold his hands out in front of him and watched as they trembled. He tapped his knee with a red rubber reflex hammer, and he shone a light in his eyes. He took a small silver pin and poked his skin.

At the end of the examination, Walter asked his doctor, "So what do you think?"

"Parkinson's. I'm sorry, Walter," his neurologist said.

"That's what I thought too," he said. Now it was official.

I met Walter when he came into the emergency room one night after cutting his leg on a mahogany end table. As he had turned the corner from the living room to his bedroom, his right leg hadn't caught up with his left. The sharp corner of the table tore into his skin and left a gash. He applied pressure but couldn't stop the bleeding.

When he arrived at the emergency room, the surgeon in his personality resurfaced. "Can you believe I spent thirty years operating on people, and here I have this little scratch on my leg and my wife makes me come to the hospital? I should have just sewed this thing up at home," he said.

His wife stood beside him with her arms folded across her chest, shaking her head in disagreement.

"Honey, it's not a scratch. And your hands aren't steady enough," she replied.

"Nonsense," he said. "My hands are plenty steady."

I caught a glimpse of his hands and noticed a significant tremor. I looked up at his wife and winked—she was right. I made sure he didn't see me wink.

I irrigated the wound for him. I opened the suture kit and set up the sterile field. "All right, I'll get the attending physician and be right back," I said.

As I turned to leave, Walter motioned for me to return.

"Will you excuse us for a moment?" Walter asked his wife.

"Walter, what are you up to?" she asked. She folded her arms across her chest.

"Please, honey," he said.

She shook her head and took a deep, disgruntled breath. "All right... fine."

Walter looked up at me, then scanned the room to be sure no one was listening. "What do you say we do this together? I call the shots—you put in the sutures?"

"I don't know if that's such a good idea, Walter." All I needed was an attending physician to lose his temper with me.

"What do you mean, not a good idea? I'm offering you something that's an opportunity of a lifetime at this stage in your career. Plus, I have twenty years of experience on your attending. Don't worry; it's easy. I'll tell you what to do. If I were a medical student, I would kill to do this. It's a win-win. You learn and I get to teach. I would do it myself if my wife would let me," he said.

The attending physician walked into the room with his long white coat, blue scrubs, and tousled hair from a busy night in the emergency room.

"All right, Walter, let's get you sutured up," he said.

"It's okay. We got it," Walter replied.

"Did he put you up to this?" He nodded in my direction.

"Don't be ridiculous; it was my idea. He's just doing his job," Walter said.

"If you're sure," the attending said.

"I'm positive." The attending left, and I could see the smile spread across Walter's face as he felt a small victory of still being in charge.

"Not that I don't trust you, but I'm going to tell you what to do, and I'm going to watch," Walter said.

"I was hoping you would," I said, laughing under my breath.

I injected local anesthetic around Walter's laceration and began suturing. He taught me to add sodium bicarbonate to the solution so it doesn't burn the skin. He taught me the importance of sterility in surgery. "Clean always beats dirty," he said. Then he showed me how to make sure my suture knots didn't slip.

But my greatest lesson was just beginning. On my sixth of twelve sutures, he turned to me and asked, "How's medical school treating you?"

"Fine... I guess," I said.

Truth is, it wasn't.

For the first time in my life, I'd contemplated quitting. I was ready to pack my bags and leave medical school. It wasn't one specific event that changed my view; it was a series: the loss of a relationship, the fatigue, the feeling I was missing out on life. I'd always been disciplined enough to put my life on hold for an end result. But lately, the light at the end of the tunnel that had once shone brightly had been a flicker and was fading fast.

"Are you in your third year of medical school?" he asked.

"Yes sir."

"Boy, that was a tough year for me. I was disillusioned with the whole process, to be honest with you—much different than I had anticipated. I was broke—not a penny to my name. My father had a farm that was not doing well, and I couldn't be there for him. It even crossed my mind to quit," Walter said.

He leaned forward and looked deep into my eyes. It seemed like an eternity. I felt uncomfortable in the silence; it was obvious he didn't. I quietly cleared my throat. I'd never told anyone that I was ready to quit. How did Walter know? Was my unhappiness that transparent?

He knew how I felt because he understood people—thirty years of taking care of patients, listening to their complaints and their fears, and seeing their emotions manifest in their illness. He'd sensed the racing of my mind and my heavy heart.

The silence ended. "But thank goodness I changed my mind. I never would have forgiven myself. I've lived a great life and helped a lot of people along the way. Now as I sit back and reflect upon my life, I realize how blessed I've been. I took care of people for a living—what a privilege. As hard as it was at times, I still miss it. I miss healing people. Sometimes you have to sacrifice. I'm proud that I gave it my all, and I never quit. And that will be important to you one day, son," he said.

While he talked, he forgot about his leg. I was finished and admiring my work.

"Good job, son—looks great," Walter said.

"I had a great teacher," I replied.

As I looked up at him, I noticed his once trembling hand was calm, and I watched a smile gently ease across his face. He looked down at me the way a proud father looks at a child. At that moment, I vowed never to quit.

Some believe that life is a series of random events and that we have little control over our lives—especially the people that enter or leave it. Not me. I believed that Walter entered my life for a specific reason. I needed him, and he was there for me.

I still do.

∽

IN THE DEEP AND DREARY WINTER OF 2009, WRITER'S BLOCK surfaced for the first time in my life. The faucet of creative flow stopped abruptly and without warning. My vision of writing a book as a gift to my children became very time-consuming. I wondered if I shouldn't just shelve the book and rethink the process again. I had a career, and I didn't need another one.

It was at this particular moment, while thumbing through the book, that I came across the chapter on Walter. In a desperate attempt to seek guidance, I tried to imagine Walter sitting across from me. I tried to remember every detail of his appearance, the sound of his voice, his mannerisms. And for a brief moment, I recalled every detail of my encounter with Walter.

And in that special moment, I vowed to see the book through and complete it. Walter would have wanted me to do so.

Walter taught me that when our life becomes cloudy, and we have drifted off track, our first tendency is to withdraw from others. He taught me to lift my head up and look around.

People will enter your life and guide you in the right direction. As long as we have an open heart and mind, people will show up and teach. But we have to be willing to learn. Good teachers need good students.

How do I know this is true?

Because when I needed Walter, he found a way to show up again.

Until Death Do Us Part

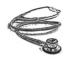

What counts in making a happy marriage
is not so much how compatible you are,
but how you deal with incompatibility.

—Leo Tolstoy

It's July of 1995, and I have successfully entered my fourth year of medical school at the Medical College of Georgia. I return to my old college campus, Emory University, to show my girlfriend, Deborah, a part of my life she has never seen. It is my attempt to fill in the gaps of life that we haven't shared together. It is Sunday, early afternoon, and the campus is empty. The libraries are crammed with students studying for exams.

I walk her around the stadium and onto the field on which I used to play soccer. I take her to my old fraternity house and into the old buildings where I studied psychology, chemistry, biology, art, and philosophy. The last stop of the tour is the Michael C. Carlos Museum. A place where I used to go to get lost in the world of art—the one place in the world where no one could find me. A place where I spent as much time as I could.

I show my girlfriend a Grecian exhibit. It is filled with dusty artifacts and pieces of ruins from the fallen empire.

"Open it," I say.

I point to a small box in the middle of the exhibit. It sits there perfectly on a small marble column and blends into the exhibit.

"I can't," she says. She looks around the room and up to the corners of the ceilings, where the security cameras watch our every move.

"If you don't, I will."

"Are you sure?" She wonders what I'm up to.

"Positive," I say.

She ducks under the red velvet ropes, walks up to the box, and slowly opens it. She begins to cry. She lifts out a diamond ring and brings it to me.

I drop down to one knee. The first teardrop turns the corner of my eye. I quietly utter the four most important words I have ever said: "Will you marry me?"

Spring of 1996

Fourth Year of Medical School

I WALKED INTO MARY'S ROOM AND NOTICED THE LIGHTS were dimmed. The darkness of night peeked through the window blinds. A small reading light above her head illuminated the book in her hands. I stood in silence and looked at her for a moment. It was my first peaceful moment of the day, and I found solace in every passing second.

Mary was in her mid-sixties and had completed chemotherapy for breast cancer. The treatment has taken its toll on her body, leaving her lethargic and weak. Her head was shaved bald, her skin tinted with a dusky hue. The dark circles under her eyes cast shadows onto her cheeks. Thin veins coursed their way just beneath her skin's fragile surface. As I looked at her, sadness filled my heart.

She was a far cry from what she'd been six months before— the fateful day that had defined the remainder of her life. The day her physician had sat across from her and said, "We received the results of your biopsy, and I am so sorry, Mary . . . it came back positive."

The cancer had taken her breast and aggressively spread throughout her body: First her lymph nodes, then her liver and lungs, and eventually into her bones. Every time her oncologists thought they were getting an edge, it showed up somewhere else. It was relentless and unforgiving. Although the treatment had targeted cancer cells, it often took healthy cells with it. It depleted her energy. Her kidneys had begun to fail, and she had recently had pneumonia. We'd tried to stabilize her medical condition so she could continue to fight.

The day I took over her care from another medical student, the student informed me about Mary's prior treatments and future plans. Before departing the student said, "Mary's such a sweet person. If you can, spend a little extra time with her. I'm sure she would enjoy the company."

When I first met Mary, she welcomed me with open arms. There were no formalities and no barriers, as if we had been friends for some time. Before I left, I asked her, "Do you need anything?"

"No, I'm fine," she said. She smiled and pointed to a chair next to her bed. "But if you want to sit and talk, you're welcome to take a seat."

I sat next to her. As we talked, some pictures across the room caught my eye. Mary noticed and looked at me.

"They're pictures of family—mostly of my husband and me."

My eye caught one picture in particular. "Do you mind if I look at it?" I asked.

"No," she said. "Be my guest."

"Is this your husband?"

"Yes," she said, smiling. "That's my husband."

In the picture, Mary looked much younger, I suspected in her early twenties, with a full head of chocolate-brown hair down to her shoulders. Her eyes squinted as if she was staring into the sun. She stood on a rock jetty, which extended out into the ocean. She and her husband were laughing.

"Are you married?" she asked.

"Yes."

"How wonderful," she said. She breathed in deeply, then exhaled slowly. "Tell me about your wife."

"Well, I've been married for a few months. My wife's a doctor too," I said. "She's in residency, and I'm finishing up school before I join her there in the fall."

"Aaah, newlyweds . . . did you meet in medical school?"

"No, we actually went to high school together."

"High school sweethearts?"

"Well, not exactly," I said. "She dated one of my friends, and I dated an acquaintance of hers."

She laughed, and her steel-blue eyes beamed even more. It was if she was returning to life right before me.

"And you?" I asked.

"Forty-six years," she said. "William and I lived the full circle of marriage. The initial stages where we learn about our spouse as we learn about ourselves, the times when we question our decisions, and try to work through our conflicts... The reality that death may tear us apart—and we may be alone."

I placed the picture back on the table, next to a photograph in a silver frame. It was a photograph of Mary and her husband on their wedding day—it was black and white but had turned a shade of sepia from age. A church with a white steeple stood in the background. William carried Mary in his arms down a long flight of stairs. From all directions, wedding guests threw rice into the air.

I thought back to my wedding day, an unseasonably warm day in February of 1996. My wedding took place in a stone cathedral with marble floors, high vaulted ceilings, and beautiful stained glass. I stood in front of God, my friends, and family, and took a leap of faith—a leap of faith in myself, my new wife, and the union of marriage.

In my life in medicine, I've witnessed how illness and other challenges in life strengthened some stable marriages and tore apart other marriages that were not structurally sound. I heard the term "we grew apart" too often. I didn't want to grow apart. I placed the picture back on the table and looked at her.

As I listened to her, I knew that marriage was a topic close to her heart. I wanted to learn from her; I sensed she knew something I didn't.

"Mary, do you mind if I ask you a personal question?" I asked.

"No," she said. "Not at all."

"What's the secret to a good marriage?"

She looked at me with unabashed honesty. "Now, that's an important question. Let me give it some thought, and I'll get back to you."

Two days later, upon morning rounds, I went back to Mary's room. I noticed things I hadn't seen before. In the center of her bedside table, there was a crystal vase filled with white tulips. Photographs of her and William surrounded the flowers: on a gondola in Venice, Italy; at the birth of their grandchild; standing on the top of a cliff overlooking a backdrop of mountains.

"When can I meet William?" I asked.

"William passed away three years ago."

"I am so sorry," I said. "I had no idea."

"It's all right," she said. "I never told you. I really don't talk about William's death much. He's still with me even though he's not physically with me. Does that make any sense?" she asked.

I nodded my head, still trying to wrap my mind around what she meant.

"He is as much a part of me in certain ways as I am. There's not a day that goes by that he's not on my mind. The day we got married, I promised to love him until death did us part. But I'm still very much in love with him."

I listened, fascinated by her attitude. She seemed sincere and grounded, not plagued with rationalization or denial.

"William is still present, not only through memories but in the legacy he left: the children, the grandchildren, our home we shared, the antiques we collected together. I see him all around me . . . he's a part of me. A part of who I am," she said. "And always will be."

She adjusted herself in bed and placed her reading glasses on the bridge of her nose. Her eyes scanned the room as if she was looking for something.

"Do you remember the other day, when you asked me the secrets to a good marriage?"

"Yes."

"Well, I wrote down a few things for you. Can you hand me that notebook?"

She pointed to a notebook on a desk across the room. I handed her the small yellow pad strung together with silver wire. At the top she had written: "The Secrets to a Good Marriage."

"If you have a moment, I'll read it to you." She began in a soft, soothing voice:

"Search for the good in your spouse. Let them know that you appreciate them. Most of us are already aware of our shortcomings in life. We need to be reminded there is good in us too. Your spouse will respond better to praise than criticism.

Give affection and love to your spouse. It's part of the human spirit. If they don't get it from you, they will be tempted to get it from others.

"The second marriage has the same challenges as the first. Before you ever decide to leave, be sure you are not equally at fault. Your personal flaws will carry over into the next relationship. Before ever trying to change your spouse, you should always work on yourself first. When you are ill, it helps to have someone you love—even if you only have their memories."

She paused and took a moment to clear her throat, then continued.

"We all need companionship. Focus on what is important: the relationship. When in doubt as to what to say—just listen. You will be much better off. Fight less and love more.

"I hope this helps you, and good luck," she said.

She ripped the paper from her notebook and handed it to me. I folded it up neatly and placed it in the right pocket of my white coat. I had every intention of taking it out that evening and putting it someplace safe, but it remained in my pocket for weeks.

One afternoon, when fumbling through my pocket, I stumbled across the folded and wrinkled paper. That night, I sat at my desk. I pushed aside my evening's work. I wrote her words in my journal so I would have them forever. I added a few other concepts she'd shared with me as well—ideas that remain with me until today. The last few words meant the most to me: "When in doubt as to what to say—just listen. Fight less and love more." To me, these words transcend marriage.

Mary once stood at the front of a church with a white steeple. In front of God, her friends, and family she took a leap of faith—in herself, in William, and the union of marriage. She looked him in the eyes, his hands in hers, and promised to love him forever. "Until death do us part," she said. It was only upon her husband's death, and during her recent illness, that she realized the greatest accomplishment of her life. She and her husband had built a marriage so strong that even death couldn't separate them.

∾

WHEN THE WORLD AROUND ME BECOMES COMPLICATED, I pull out Mary's "Secrets to a Good Marriage" and review them. I still find something new, or an idea to think about, depending on where I am in my life. In their simplicity lies great value. It provides a foundation of thought for me, and then I find myself writing and adding to her list as I continue to grow in my relationship with my wife.

It seems like yesterday that I stood in front of my friends and family and promised to love my wife forever and to stay with her until death did us part. I recall the words *death* and *forever* seeming so distant. Now, on my seventeenth year of marriage, I am astonished how quickly time passes. And how *death* and *forever* have taken on real meaning—no longer existing as intangible words. I find great satisfaction in watching my relationship with my wife evolve and grow.

I now understand what Mary meant about the life she built with William. When I look around me . . . I see my wife in everything: in our home, in the life we have built together, in the eyes of our children. It took Mary's wisdom mixed with my own experience to understand. But now I do.

And it remains true; Mary's words continue to transcend marriage for me. We would all be much better off if we listened to one another, fought less, and loved more.

Be Present

I stood staring at this little girl, swaddled tightly in
soft blankets, with bright blue eyes and pink flushed
skin. Her small hand wrapped around my thumb.
I held her close to my face and placed a kiss upon her
forehead. I thought to myself, I will always take care
of you and love you ... no matter what.

June 16, 2002—the day our first daughter was born

"Push!" I say. "Push!"

It's a sweltering summer evening at Grady Memorial Hospital in August of 1996. I am in my internship year of medical residency on a rotation in Obstetrics and Gynecology.

My palms are sweaty, my heart races, and adrenaline pumps through my body—every physician is nervous the first time they deliver a baby on their own.

Maria arches her back even further and breathes in deeply. Her rosy cheeks are filled with air. Her dark hair spills onto her chest. Sweat beads up on her forehead and rolls down her temples. She exhales loudly, letting out a groan.

A nurse stands to my left and offers Maria support. She is braced in stirrups, but the epidural makes her legs feel like jelly.

"One more time," I say. "I need one more push, and your baby will be born." I see the baby's hair as he is crowning.

Maria begins to cry.

"Maria, stay with me now. One more push and that's it."

She takes three deep breaths in rapid succession. She purses her lips and sucks in one final big, deep breath. She opens her mouth and lets out every ounce of air in her lungs.

The baby glides his way into my hands. He is warm and slippery. I place one hand behind the base of his neck and cup the small of his back with the other. I bring him close to my chest. I suction his nose and mouth with a blue rubber syringe. He takes in his first breath of life and lets out a loud cry.

I hold him against my face and whisper into his ear, "Happy birthday, little boy … happy birthday."

Spring 1996

Fourth Year of Medical School

SEAN SAT IN AN OAK ROCKING CHAIR BY THE WINDOW OF HIS hospital room and glided slowly back and forth so he could feel the warmth of the morning sun against his face. His scant dark hair was combed neatly off his forehead, and his skin smelled of lotion. His thick cotton pajamas engulfed his withering body, and a blanket lay across his lap to help prevent his frequent and sudden chills.

His current appearance was a far cry from last spring. For sixty years, Sean had led a clean life. He'd eaten well, he exercised daily, and he didn't smoke or drink alcohol. He was in better shape than anyone he knew his age—he did everything he could to keep healthy.

At his last college reunion, the women had come up to him saying, "Well, you haven't aged a day since the last time I saw you." He always blushed when they complimented him.

One September morning, after breakfast, a horrendous cough had rattled his body. Never had he coughed so hard. He'd swirled some cough medicine with codeine, but it didn't touch the cough. It resided deep within his lungs. That afternoon he'd spit up blood into his handkerchief. He'd called his wife, Nancy, and told her of the day's events. She'd rushed him to the hospital.

When an X-ray had revealed a suspicious area at the top of his right lung, the emergency room doctor had ordered a CT of his chest. It revealed more suspicious areas. A lung specialist had placed a tube down his throat and come up with a sample of the tissue. A pathologist had sliced up the tissue and studied it under a microscope.

His lung specialist had broken the news. "I'm sorry, Sean, but you have lung cancer."

"Lung cancer? But I never smoked a cigarette in my life."

"I know," the doctor said. "There is nothing you could have done to prevent this—you are the exception to the rule on this terrible disease."

That, for Sean, was the hardest part to understand. "How do we treat it?" Sean had asked.

"We can try chemotherapy and radiation, but it's inoperable. One of the tests showed that it has spread into your liver and to your stomach. The bone scan showed it has spread into your bones."

A solemn look had spread across Sean's face and his voice had quivered. "How long do I have?"

"Three to six months."

"That's it? That's all?"

"I'm so sorry."

I met Sean at the latter part of his life. He was a week away from hospice care. He focused on trying to rebuild his strength, to lead a more functional life, in his few remaining months. I tried to alleviate his pain.

As I looked around his hospital room, it was evident that many people loved him. Flowers covered the countertops, the windowsill, even the top of an old heater. There were pink lilies and blue hydrangeas and magenta tulips. There were handwritten notes and poems attached to the walls with scotch tape. There was a small oil painting on his nightstand that leaned up against the wall, from a French artist he had befriended. And there were lots of pictures—pictures of his children, his wife, and his friends.

The objects around him meant something to him; each represented a piece of a puzzle. When put together, they told the story of his life.

He had a constant stream of visitors: colleagues, family members, people from church, old schoolmates, old friends, and new friends. The nurses tried to limit the amount of visitors, but he resisted.

"I'll go to bed soon, I promise; just let him in," he would say.

It was clear he had made an impact on the world one person at a time.

I met all three of Sean's children on different occasions: His youngest son was a banker; his daughter, a stay-at-home mother; and his eldest son, a preacher. I commented to Sean on how well-adjusted they seemed.

"Do you have any children?" he asked.

"No," I said. "We're trying to find the perfect time."

He coughed to clear his throat and spit weakly into a handkerchief. "I hate to kill the suspense for you, but do you want to know the truth?"

"Yes."

He smiled. "There is never a perfect time, son. If you are thinking about it and you want children, you're ready."

"Do you mind if I ask you a question?" I asked.

"No."

"How did you raise such good children?"

At the time, my wife and I were thinking about starting a family. But I wondered how I would achieve balance in the midst of a challenging career. It was no secret; doctors often make poor spouses and parents. I didn't want to fail as a parent, so I leaned on Sean for advice.

He rocked in his chair and then paused for a moment until the chair stopped moving. He raised a coffee cup to his lips and took a sip. His hand trembled, and the coffee swirled around the rim without spilling.

"The key to being a good parent is to be present for them," he said, and then he paused to make sure I had heard him. "Be present for them."

He laid his head back in the rocking chair. "I don't know if you know this, but my father was a doctor—an old-school family practitioner."

"I didn't know."

"Well, we grew up in a small town in Indiana, and he was the only physician in town. He delivered babies, performed surgery, and took care of children. He worked from the moment he got out of bed until it was dark. And when he got home the phone would ring—he was off to make house calls with his little black bag and stethoscope. In the rain, in the snow—and if he couldn't get there by car, he walked."

He relaxed in his chair. His mind journeyed back in time.

"He was a good man, but he put his practice before his family. He was never with us. My mom raised us. And children need a father figure in their life. I vowed to never do that. I decided I would be the father figure that I never had," he said.

He looked at me. "The key is to leave the work at the office. I don't care what you do for a living. If you're not home, your children will notice—they will suffer."

He took a small pillow and wedged it behind the base of his back for support. "Children need your time and love more than anything else. Turn off the television. Put down the newspaper. Get down on the floor, to your children's level, and absorb yourself in their world: Color, paint, and be present—and not just in body. Give them your mind and your heart. They deserve that."

∾

TO THIS DAY, WHEN MY LIFE DRIFTS OFF TRACK, AND WORK spills over into my family time, I hear the words of Sean: "Be present." His words remind me to cherish the precious times with my children. There will come a day, far too soon, where their own life will take priority over their time with me. Life runs away far too fast.

Just recently, I let work spill over into my life again. The balance of my life was disrupted. It started simply enough. I'd brought home a few things from work. As all bad habits go, more were soon to follow. I dictated charts and read journal articles. I asked my family to be quiet while I worked. My daughter said nothing but looked at me. I saw she was hurt. I could tell by the curl of her lip and the water welling up in her eyes.

There are few things that pull at a father's heartstrings more than to watch the feelings of disappointment spread across a young child's face. Sean's voice immediately lit up my mind: "Be present."

I put down my work.

I thought about my young daughters, and the times when they are most fulfilled—when my wife and I sit in the playroom or lie down on the floor beside them. When we take the time to join them among the Barbie dolls, princess costumes, crayons, and shaggy brown teddy bears. We talk about their day, and we play and laugh together. We let go of our busy lives and enter their world. I see the joy in their eyes and the smiles on their faces. In these moments, I understand exactly what Sean meant.

And when I follow his advice, I am never disappointed.

Letting Go

Communication. It is not only
the essence of being human but
also a vital property of life.

—JOHN A. PIERCE

It's my fourth year of medical school in the spring of 1996, and I am at the tail end of a rotation at Savannah Memorial Hospital. It was a busy night on the trauma service, and when I return to my room in the morning, I find myself unable to sleep. The events of the evening keep playing through my mind.

I decide to go down by the river—a peaceful setting with quaint restaurants and great views. I walk down the cobblestone streets and watch the boats drift in the harbor. I eventually settle into a small café. A soft spring rain begins to fall, making the patrons of the patio seek shelter. A father and son settle in at the table next to me. They are returning from an early church service. Their conversation quickly turns toward the son's relationship with his girlfriend.

"So, what do you think? Is she the one?" the father asks.

"I don't know ... maybe?"

*"What do you mean, maybe? She's beautiful; she's smart . . .
she comes from a good family. What else do you want?" His father leans closer to him. "You know your mom and I would love
for you to settle down. We want grandchildren."*

"I know. But I'm not sure I can trust her."

*"What?" The father's mood changes. "Do you think she
cheated on you?"*

*"No, Dad." The son laughs. "It's nothing like that. But the
other day I asked her if she had any regrets—anything in life she
would have done differently. And she looked me right in the eyes
and told me no."*

"So what?" the father replies.

*"Well, Dad, you always told me to never trust anybody who
says they have no regrets."*

"I did? When did I say that?"

Spring of 1996

Fourth Year of Medical School

A S I WALKED INTO CHARLIE'S ROOM, THE FIRST THING I
noticed was its simplicity. No flowers, no pictures, no get-
well cards—just Charlie.

The only sound was an air-conditioning unit quietly buzz-
ing in the corner. The windows of his room were closed, and

the curtains were drawn shut. A dim light from a small lamp in the corner provided the only hint of warmth.

Charlie was a New York City police officer who had transferred to Georgia after a fair-skinned girl from Savannah had stolen his heart. After thirty years of service, he'd reached his goal of staying until age fifty, and left on top. He had felt the walls of New York City closing in on him, and sensed the criminals were becoming more dangerous. He'd escaped danger too many times, and felt an ominous sign stirring within him that luck couldn't carry him the distance. He knew he needed a change.

He was six foot three with dark ruddy skin and a broken nose. "A few times a crook tried to take a swing at me and I forgot to duck," he said, pointing proudly to his nose. He made sure you knew that in the end he'd won.

I looked at the large bandage across his abdomen. It was obvious that luck hadn't had his back this time. The elephant in the room was sitting right in front of me.

"So tell me about it," I began.

"Well, sometimes in my off-duty hours, I work at a club doing security. The other night these two guys began talking trash. I step in the middle—just to try to tell them to settle down and cool their heads—when one pulls out a knife and stabs me. Can you believe that? People just have no respect for human life anymore," he said.

"What did you do?"

"What do you think I did? I disarmed him, and then I taught him a lesson about why you don't stab a police officer. I would imagine he's somewhere in this hospital too . . . I left my old job because I thought it was becoming too dangerous, and here I am in the safest job I know, and I end up getting stabbed."

The next morning on rounds, I informed him that he was free to leave that afternoon.

The nurse entered. "Would you like some pain medicine?"

"Nah, I'm all right," he said, pausing just long enough to look at her before returning his eyes to the newspaper.

"By the way," I asked. "Where did you live in New York?"

He laughed. "Most people here in Savannah think I'm from Boston."

We talked about the great city of New York: the plays, the restaurants, the passion for sports, and the resilience of the people.

He became more reserved, and his voice softened. "Do you have any regrets, Doctor?"

"I'm sure I do; don't we all?" I thought for a moment. "I think most of mine have to do with relationships," I said.

He shook his head in agreement.

"Yeah, I understand that. I know I have regrets. I just got off the phone with my wife. I'm leaving for New York in the morning to find my son."

My mind raced, thinking about the possible scenarios. I sensed the wrenching of his heart.

"Is he okay?"

"God, I hope so," he said. "When I was a child, my father was tough on me and my brother—he liked the belt, if you know what I mean."

I nodded my head and listened with sympathetic ears.

"It's all right; it's been many years. But I vowed to never be like him. I decided to create strict rules so that I would never have to lay a hand on my child. I told him firmly that if he ever broke the law, he was out of the house. Period. I couldn't accept being a police officer and him disrespecting my profession or me as a father."

He looked down toward his feet.

"Then one day I get a call from my captain. 'Hey, Charlie, we got your son down here. He and some friends just got picked up for vandalism and burglary.' I lost it. I told him to lock my son up, and then tell him that he is not welcome in my house anymore. It tore me up, having my son in jail. But I didn't know what to do. I felt if I backed down now he would never respect me. And when he got home, I threw him out of the house. He cried and cried, but I wouldn't let him back. He tried to contact me, but I wouldn't go back on my word."

He wiped his hand across his brow.

"Since that day I haven't been the same person. I miss my son. Tomorrow, I'm going to New York. I'm going to find him and tell him how sorry I am."

Every hint of the bravado he'd once hidden behind was gone.

"Hey, Doctor, when you have children, love them no matter what—love them. Nothing should ever come between a parent and a child."

He looked at me with the eyes of a broken soul.

"Nothing … "

∞

I OFTEN WONDER IF CHARLIE FOUND HIS SON, AND WHAT HE did say when he saw him for the first time after that separation. Or maybe he didn't talk at all. Maybe he just embraced his son and promised himself silently never to let go.

Charlie taught me about letting go of regrets. You don't need a brush with mortality to ask for forgiveness. You need a light heart and a willingness to rise above.

Now that I have two beautiful daughters, I focus on loving them unconditionally—no matter what obstacles we may encounter. I find comfort in knowing that Charlie would be proud.

Charlie was right. "Nothing should ever come between a parent and a child."

I tell my children every day of my life that I love them. I believe they need to hear it… almost as much as I need to tell them.

Having the Courage to Open Your Heart

A light heart lives longer.

—Irish Proverb

It's a gray winter day of my third year of medical school in 1994. I wait outside the office of my former medical school professor, Dr. Weidman, glancing frequently at the clock above the doorway. I wipe my sweaty palms on my pants, hoping to hide my nervousness. As I look out the window, I see him hobble up the stairs to his office.

He walks past me briskly, a briefcase in his right hand and a stack of mail in his left hand. He opens the door and motions for me to enter. I sit across the desk from him. I stare at the rows of books, the gold-framed diplomas on his walls, the academic awards he has received.

"How can I help you?" he asks. He leans forward on his desk and braces himself with his elbows lying flat on the table and his hands held close together. His normal casual demeanor is absent. Suddenly, I feel the warmth of the spotlight of his attention on me. I feel intimidated. I silently wonder why I made

the decision to make the appointment in the first place. He seems very busy. I feel embarrassed.

All the clear thoughts in my head, present only moments ago, have vanished without warning. I feel the need to clear my throat. "I'm sorry to bother you," I say. "I'm just having a hard time right now, and I need your opinion."

"About what?" he asks.

"Do you ever have students that have one vision of medicine and then it turns out to be quite different ... maybe it wasn't at all what they expected?" I ask.

He nods and leans back in his chair.

I look him in the eyes. "Well, any advice?"

"Yes. Create your own vision."

And without missing a beat, he picks up his mail and starts sorting through it.

Fall of 1997

Second Year of Medical Residency

ISAAC WAS A TEACHER AT HEART. HE PACED THE FLOOR OF A grand auditorium and taught college students the finer details of the world's architecture. Slide by slide, he took students to places in the world they had never been—from the buildings of the Roman Empire to the ruins of Greece. His passion was evident in his voice, his enthusiasm contagious.

He used his hands to convey his message the way a masterful conductor leads a string section of an orchestra.

His passion for architecture spilled over into other areas of his life: drawing, writing, and traveling. He was in his late eighties with beautiful tanned skin, silver flowing hair, and bushy eyebrows. The sun ages most of us, but it had nourished his skin.

One spring morning as he got dressed for work, he felt an electrical jolt in his arm and down his leg. As he spoke, the words came out jumbled. He tried to stand, but his leg gave out beneath him. He fell on the floor and curled up like a baby.

His stroke took many things away from him—the ability to walk, the ability to use his left hand while telling a story— but for Isaac the inability to eat was the cruelest. The stroke had paralyzed the muscles that divert the food in the right direction. We sent him for a swallowing test. Every time Isaac swallowed food, it ended up in his lungs instead of his stomach. So I had to place a tube through his nose into his stomach to make sure the food went to the right place.

The next morning on rounds he asked me, "How about a little pudding, Doctor?"

He was drawing on a napkin with a coffee stain in the center.

"Isaac, you know we can't give you anything by mouth. You could aspirate and get very sick," I said.

He handed me the napkin—a silhouette of a man in black ink holding a loaf of bread. At the top it said, "A hungry man dreams of loaves of bread."

"How about just a little, then?" he asked.

"I'm so sorry, Isaac, but I can't," I replied.

Isaac's love for food had begun when he was a child growing up in a small town in Greece. Food was more than nourishment for his body; it was an experience. He loved the taste, the texture, and the smell. He sat back in his bed and told me about the times he would sit for hours with friends. He remembered each topic of conversation, the food, the wine, and the people around him. But most of all the company. Food had just enhanced the experience.

That afternoon, I sat at a long table surrounded by Isaac's caregivers. The physical therapist said, "He is coming along nicely, but he keeps trying to sneak food."

"Yeah, I saw him trying to steal a cookie off another patient's plate at lunch today," the occupational therapist chimed in.

All eyes turned on me. "How about you, Dr. Kelly?"

I couldn't snitch. I couldn't turn him in. "I'll talk to him," I said. "I'll talk to him." I didn't lie, but I didn't exactly tell the truth.

Immediately after the meeting, I went into Isaac's room with firm intentions to scold him.

"You have to take this seriously. You have got to try to stop eating food—at least until you can swallow properly," I said.

"Yeah, I know, I know," he said as he shrugged his shoulders. He quickly changed the subject.

"Hey, what do you say—when I get out of here, you and I go to Manuel's Tavern for a drink?" he said.

"What?"

"Manuel's Tavern. It's this place I go with a group of friends. We meet there and discuss different topics. We talk mostly politics, but we talk about other things as well: civil rights, city corruption, and ways to make the world better. We have beers, we laugh—you should join me. You can be my guest," he said.

"Fine. You stop trying to sneak food, and I'll join you at Manuel's Tavern," I said. To be honest, I didn't plan on going. I never thought he would take me up on it.

Doctors are taught to keep their distance from patients. We're taught to safeguard our hearts yet to try to remain compassionate and empathetic. It's a concept that is sound in theory but difficult to implement on a consistent basis. We're told it affects our decision-making if we get too close. We need to stay focused—in the eye of the storm. If we get emotionally involved it can cloud our vision, and we won't make clear decisions for our patients. By staying distant, we better serve our patients.

Isaac's invitation was all but forgotten until one bright, sunny morning when he was being discharged from the hospital. A nurse pushed him out in a wheelchair, and he motioned for her to stop. He turned his head toward me over his shoulder.

"So next Wednesday, six, at Manuel's," he said.

I had made a deal with him. Maybe just this once, I would bend my rules. "All right, a deal's a deal. I'll see you there," I said. I smiled and laughed under my breath.

The next Wednesday, I found myself winding through the roads of the eclectic neighborhood of the Virginia-Highlands area of North Atlanta. The streets are lined with overhanging trees, antique stores, art galleries, and pubs with a history. I soon arrived at Isaac's favorite—Manuel's tavern, named after Manuel Maloof. Manuel was a local favorite who knew where he stood in life and wasn't afraid to share his political views with anyone who cared to listen.

Manuel was a local icon, his character larger than life. He was a staunch Democrat who had a fondness for John F. Kennedy and people who served their country: police officers, servicemen, and firemen mostly. His passion in life was conversations—about politics. His silver hair and his big smile were disarming. But he was a man of passion. His heart was enormous, but his temper carried a short fuse.

When I walked in through the door, the first person I saw was Manuel himself. He stood at the long oak bar surrounded by five people sitting on bar stools. They all sat on the edge of their seats, listening to him talk about politics.

He gave one guy a hard time. "You got to be kidding me," he said. "Do you actually believe that?" I saw everyone around him laugh.

I entered the back room of the rustic tavern. On my way, I looked at the pictures of the many political figures that had stopped by to say hello to Manuel when in town: President Bill Clinton, President Jimmy Carter, and Vice President Al Gore.

I sat with a group of men I didn't know and my friend Isaac. He sat in a wheelchair, still weak from his hospital stay, with a blanket wrapped around his shoulders to keep his frail body warm. The air was filled with the smell of stale beer and cigar smoke. There had been many attempts at solving the world's problems at this establishment. Some better than others—it depended upon how much the patrons had to drink.

I turned to Isaac. "Are you all right?"

He looked around the room, taking it all in. "I'm great. It's good to be back here. It's great to be back in the world."

He placed his hand on my knee. I placed my hand on his.

"Thank you for coming with me, my friend," he said.

"It's good to be here, Isaac."

And I got a glimpse into Isaac's world. We talked about life and politics. We talked about his career. We talked about how much he loved his family, how proud he was of his daughter. And we became better friends. If I hadn't opened my heart and let him in, I would have missed out on a great friendship.

He turned to me and whispered in my ear, "Do you remember when I first talked to you about coming to Manuel's with me?"

I did. I quickly looked down to my shoes, avoiding eye contact. I felt embarrassed.

"I know what you were thinking. It's all right. It's natural. You don't want to get emotionally involved with every patient. It could hurt you in the end. I understand that."

He paused and looked around the room—at his friends, the bar patrons, the bartenders.

"But if you close yourself off to people, how are you ever going to learn?"

My eyes drifted from my shoes back to his kind eyes.

"You are in a position to touch the hearts of others. If you build up emotional barriers around yourself, no one can get in. It's not always them that loses—it's you too. Sure, there will be times when you're hurt, but it's better than closing yourself off to the world around you. Let people in—and you will grow too."

At the end of the evening, I wheeled him out to his car for a friend to take him home. I put my arms around his neck, my cheek to his.

"Let's keep in touch," he said.

I nodded. "All right," I said. "And thank you."

I had every intention of keeping in touch with Isaac, but that was the last time I saw my friend, and the last time I saw Manuel Maloof—both have left this world. I miss them both; the world was a better place with them in it.

Isaac taught me that night to open my heart to others, even if I might get hurt. I've been trying to keep it open ever since.

∾

WHILE WRITING THIS BOOK, I RETURNED TO MANUEL'S TAVERN. Many years had passed since I was last there with Isaac. I hoped my presence would rekindle my memories of my time with Isaac, and infuse some of my dear friend's wisdom back into me.

I drove down the tangled streets of North Highland Avenue, and was pleased to see the overhanging trees still stood proud, and many of the antique galleries, art stores, and old pubs remained. Manuel's Tavern still sits on the corner, as if time stood still.

Upon entering, I decided to walk first to the room where Isaac and I had talked. The same brick floors and brick walls remained. The photographs of the politicians, the painting of John F. Kennedy, the memorabilia from policemen and firemen still hung on the walls.

At the table that Isaac and I had shared sat a diverse group of people—some in their early thirties and a few in their late seventies. Some were blue collar and others wore suits. If you plucked them out of Manuel's and put them in another environment, I suspect that none of them would share the time of day, much less carry on a conversation. But Manuel had had a way of bringing people together and transcending economic classes and social barriers. He knew all along that politics and drinking and a general concern for the world provoked thought. It made people talk. And conversation—but more importantly communicating—was his oxygen. And as he opened up, everyone around him did too.

As I stood there, a general sense of easiness graced my presence—as if all the thoughts of my mind cleared. A sense of serenity and complacency filled me. Nothing seemed to press me to leave, and I became absorbed in the moment. I thought about my time with Isaac, and I felt closer to him.

I walked into the main room and sat down at the bar. At the top left, there was a small wooden encasement with a silver vase. Above it, a folded American flag sat. In the vase were the ashes of Manuel Maloof. How perfect, I thought. I smiled knowing that, if given the choice, Manuel would rather be nowhere else.

I looked around the room and marveled at how little had changed. Maybe some things are so good they don't need to be changed. They transcend time. Isaac once told me to open my heart to others so that I could learn. Maybe some principles are so good and pure that they stand the test of time too.

In fact, I know it's true. I'm certain of it.

Finding Purpose

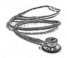

As my pediatrician walks into the room, it is as if God himself has graced me with his presence. His starched white coat, tender demeanor, and soft-spoken voice make me feel that while I am with him, nothing in the world can harm me. The simple touch of his warm hand makes me feel better, long before he listens to my heart or looks in my ears.

I know at that moment what I want to do for the rest of my life—I want to make others feel the way he makes me feel.

At that moment, I decide to become a doctor.

—WINTER, 1974

It is mid-season for the Emory Eagles soccer team in the fall of 1991. It is five minutes before game time; we are warmed up and mentally prepared to take on Washington University from St. Louis. As I walk toward the field, a man approaches me. He is tall and wiry with blond thinning hair and a big smile. He reaches his hand out to me. His large hand engulfs mine.

"I wanted to meet you," he says. "I'm Sonny Carter. I used to play soccer here many years ago. And when I watch you play,

*I see a little bit of myself. It brings back a lot of good memories."
A broad grin spreads across his face. "Good luck today." And
with that he pats me on the back and walks over and into the
crowd of people in the stands.*

*I stand for a moment in awe. Sonny Carter is an icon. To me
he is larger than life. By his early forties he became a physician,
played professional soccer, and became a Top Gun fighter pilot.
He is now an astronaut. There is nothing in life that seems too
big of a challenge for him—nothing he fears.*

*I play my heart out in that game, knowing Sonny is watching.
After the game, I look for him but can't find him. When I head to
the locker room, I see him leaning against a railing, looking at a
wall of pictures of former All-Americans. His back is facing me.
I rush up to talk to him.*

"Sonny?" I say.

*He turns toward me. We talk about his time at Emory, his
professional soccer stint, his life in medicine, his time as a fighter
pilot, and his venture into space.*

*"There is nothing like it," he says. "Looking down on earth—
it's the most beautiful thing your eyes will ever see." He looks at
me and reads my thoughts. "Even better than you're imagining
right now."*

*"If you don't mind me asking, how did you accomplish so
much?" I ask.*

*He pauses. It's clear he's been asked the same question be-
fore. "For me, it was never about accomplishments. I just do the
things in life that inspire me, and I try to do my best at those
things. I trust the rest to take care of itself."*

As I look at him, he senses I am looking for more.

"There's no real secret. Just do the things in life that inspire you. The accomplishments will come."

In early April, only eight months later, I walk out on my doorstep to pick up the newspaper. On the front page is a picture of Sonny Carter. He died in a plane crash in Brunswick, Georgia, on a commercial airplane flight on April 5, 1991. At that moment, I feel a small part of me die with him. I respect him that much.

In 1993, the Sonny Carter Elementary School opens in his hometown of Macon, Georgia. When looking for a motto, they come up with "To Challenge the Edge of the Universe." How appropriate, I think.

Until I realize the universe doesn't stand a chance against Sonny.

Late Fall of 1997

Second Year of Medical Residency

I WALKED INTO HARRISON'S ROOM AND FOUND AN EMPTY BED. I went to his favorite place—a faded gray park bench outside the hospital—hoping to find him there. He shared with me that he would go there to think and to escape the loneliness of the hospital. I smiled when I saw him from a distance.

He sat alone under a tall dogwood tree. The empty branches of the tree gently swayed with the wind. Winter loomed around the corner. The cold didn't seem to bother him; he was in his own world. He was focused on writing in his journal, and as I approached, he paused and patted the bench next to him, inviting me to sit.

"I never dreamed of having a journal before I got sick," he said. "Now I can't imagine my life without one." He sat in silence for a moment, and his mood turned reflective. "Doctor, if you had to pick one fear, what would it be?"

"Sharks," I blurted out. Then I looked back at the hospital behind me, taking in all I'd seen within its walls. "Maybe living in pain ... followed by dying."

"You have to pick one," he said.

"All right then, dying," I said.

"Yeah," he said. "Me too."

At the age of thirty-three, Harrison led a demanding life. The rumors swirled around his office that in a few months he would be a partner in his law firm. He pressed on. He awoke before the sun rose and found his way home late in the evenings long after the sun fell. His weekends were spent catching up on the work that rolled in late in the week. When he finished, he spent the rest of his time with his wife and children. There was little time left for him.

One morning, Harrison sat in front of the bathroom mirror. He combed his blond, thinning hair and brushed his teeth. He lathered his face with shaving cream. When he shaved under his chin, he cut himself. As he applied tissue to control the bleeding, he felt a lump—it was firm and round. He thought nothing of it and left for work.

Three weeks later he went to play basketball. He'd played on the same team for years with a group of friends. Harrison was normally one of the best players. This game he was tired and lethargic; it was evident in his play.

A teammate asked him if he was all right.

"I'm fine," he said. "I've been working too hard. We'll get them next time."

That night his wife lay next to him in bed with her head against his chest. Her hand brushed across a nodule on his chest.

"My God, Harrison, what is this?" she asked.

"I don't know. I've had a few of these lately."

"A few—and you didn't tell me?"

"I didn't want to worry you," he said.

"Tomorrow, you're going to the doctor."

"But, I have a deposition—"

She cut him off in midsentence. "I don't care—tomorrow," she said. And that was that.

The next day, Harrison went to his doctor's office. Harrison told him about the lump while shaving, his fatigue playing basketball, the nodule on his chest. The doctor felt the mass.

A concerned look spread across his face. The doctor sent him to the hospital for blood work, X-rays, and a biopsy of the mass along his clavicle. That night, he dreamed he was dying of lymphoma. The word had never entered his mind before, but somehow he just knew.

Harrison was right. The biopsy confirmed his fear.

I met Harrison after his lymphoma had spread. Radiation and chemotherapy had slowed the progress of the disease but drained his energy. He was weak and thin. His muscular frame

had withered. His hair had fallen out. He seemed depressed—
a man of few words. I tried to make conversation, but he was
distant. His thoughts focused on his disease.

Two mornings later, I walked into his room. He had a smile
across his face.

"How's your day going?" I asked.

"Wonderful," he said. "I just retired."

"Really?" I said. "You seem awfully young to be retired." I
hoped he hadn't made a hasty decision based on his recent turn
of events.

"Well, I don't mean that I'm done working," he said. "I'm
just done being a lawyer."

"Have you told your firm that yet?"

"No, but I've told my wife, and she supports me. I'll tell
them next week. I just can't do it anymore," he said.

"Why now?" I asked.

"Well, my illness provides me with certain freedoms. Like
the ability to say no—freedoms I've never experienced. The
upside of illness is clarity of thought—the gray areas of life become more clear, more black and white."

"Were you ever happy being a lawyer?" I asked.

"Not really. I became a lawyer for all the wrong reasons. My
dad was a lawyer, my brother was a lawyer—I felt I didn't have
a choice. I didn't want to disappoint or shake the family tree,"
he said. "I did the job, but the truth is, I wasn't happy."

"What do you think you'll do now?" I asked.

"I don't know for sure. Maybe something in nonprofit…
maybe I'll become a doctor," he said, and smiled.

"Well, it's never too late, you know."

He laughed, and then the smile slowly disappeared from his face.

"I just know that life is too short to be doing something I don't love. I would rather have less in my life than spend my time wishing I were somewhere else. I don't want to live my life trading my time for money—not now, not anymore."

"Is that your biggest fear?" I asked.

"No," he said, shaking his head. "My biggest fear is still dying." He paused and then stole a quick, deep breath. "My second is that I will live and will end up wealthy, but broke and empty on the inside."

~

FROM TIME TO TIME, I AM ASKED TO GIVE A LECTURE TO students about the career choice of becoming a physician. At a lecture at Emory University in 2009, a young student from a leadership organization raised her hand. She waited patiently in the last row.

I had been fielding the usual questions that evening: Can you get over feeling queasy at the sight of blood? How do you function with the lack of sleep? Do you think you will one day be working for the government? And my least favorite, but which surfaces every lecture—How much money do doctors make? But her question was different.

"If you had to do it all over again, would you?" she asked.

"Great question," I said. I paced the center of the room and gave her question ample thought. After careful consideration I responded, "Yes, I would."

And when she heard my answer, her face lit up.

On the way home that evening, I thought of what Sonny Carter once told me: "Just do the things in life that inspire you. The accomplishments will come." And for a moment, the world around me made sense. I had chosen to become a physician that day in the pediatrician's office. He had inspired me. I was one of the lucky ones. I found my purpose early in life, and it turned into a career. I had done exactly what Sonny had advised me to. I felt proud.

As I thought more, I realized that my decision to write came from the same place in my mind. I write because it interests me and inspires me. Simple as that.

My encounter with Harrison reminded me that I was on the correct path. And reassurance is a welcome companion in life. He also reminded me that it is never too late to change your mind. That was important for me too. It's nice to have the thought of a lifeboat floating around in the sea of your mind just in case the weather turns on you. So far, the waters have remained calm.

The young student in the last row led me to reevaluate my choice of career. The true litmus test is to ask yourself: "If you had to do it all over again, would you?" I've asked myself that question many times since then, and I've always come to the same conclusion.

You bet I would.

In Search of Happiness

I don't know what your destiny will be,
but one thing I do know: the only ones among
you who will be really happy are those
who have sought and found how to serve.

—ALBERT SCHWEITZER

It's the end of a rotation in our first year of medical residency in 1997, and a few medical residents decide to go to dinner to celebrate. We sit around and talk about life. The conversation turns toward dreams. Our life is on hold during medical residency, so we live for our dreams.

"If you could live anywhere, where would it be?" asks a resident.

"California," says one.

"Why?"

"The weather's perfect."

"How about you?" he asks a young female resident.

"Seattle."

"Why Seattle?"

"It's got mountains and ocean."

"Yeah, but it rains too much," another resident says.

"How about you?" he asks me. "Where would you want to live?"

"Right here," I say. "I'm staying here."

"Why? You could live anywhere," he says.

"Because it's my home. It's where I'm happy," I say.

We all look at one another for a moment and embrace the silence. Then suddenly he looks up at me.

"I wish I had a place like that," he says.

And then I think about the beauty of California and Seattle, and my mind wonders if I'm making the right decision.

Spring of 1998

Second Year of Medical Residency

THE DOGWOODS WERE IN FULL BLOOM IN THE SPRING OF 1998 in Atlanta, Georgia. The sweet smell of nectar filled the air, and a gentle breeze nudged the clouds across the pale-blue sky. The tall oak trees cast shadows onto the front façade of Emory University Hospital.

I walked through the large doors of the hospital and entered the formal entrance. French antiques, Italian marble, and oil portrait paintings of past presidents lined the walls. As I walked down the narrow hallway into the main hospital, it felt like I had left one world and entered another. A world where the mood became somber, the pain was palpable, and the scent of spring was replaced by the smell of sickness.

Within moments, I saw many faces of grief.

I saw a tall man with dark-brown skin and deep lines in his forehead. He was leaning against one of the walls just outside of the waiting room. Years of construction work had taken a visible toll on his body. His back was braced against the wall for support; his head was tilted up toward the ceiling. He had just lost his son in a car accident. He waited patiently for further instructions—where to pick up the body and how to get it to the funeral home. He smoked a cigarette underneath a sign that said, "Please, No Smoking." He looked hopeless and in a great deal of pain. I simply didn't have the heart to tell him to put it out.

As I turned the corner, I saw the woman with the faded jeans and plaid shirt in the waiting room outside the Intensive Care Unit. She had been there for days. She sat forward with her arms across her knees. She drank stale, cold coffee from a white Styrofoam cup. She was afraid to leave the hospital for a shower or a night of good rest. Her husband was losing his battle against pancreatic cancer. Any moment away could be his last. We all understood.

On morning rounds, I stopped by Andrew's room. Andrew was recovering from a hip replacement. He was a distin-guished-looking man with a bronzed face and silver hair care-fully parted to the side. He was clean-shaven, and a light scent of aftershave filled the room. As I scanned his chart, I noticed he was reading a book—*The Art of Happiness*. I watched his eyes scan the pages and consume them.

"Hey, Dr. Kelly, I didn't hear you come in." He pointed to a chair beside his seat. "Come, sit down."

He adjusted his pillow and laid a red ribbon across the page to mark his spot. He took off his glasses. He pulled the book close to his chest, against his heart. He saw me shoot a glance at the book.

He turned the front cover toward me. "A friend of mine got it for me. He said the hospital was a lonely place, and I needed something to keep me company when visiting hours were over." He smiled. "He was right."

"Learn anything new?"

"You know, I believe I did. I have always been fascinated by what motivates people. What makes us tick? I remember learning in high school about Darwin—he thought it was survival. And then I learned about Freud in college."

"Sex, right?"

"Exactly." He looked at the cover of the book. "The Dalai Lama—he believes we are motivated by the pursuit of happiness—everything we do is a direct effort to achieve happiness. After reading this, I believe he is right."

I stood up beside him. I put on beige latex gloves and snapped them around my wrists.

"Happiness, that's it? That's what motivates us?" I asked.

"Yes, we begin to look for change in our life when our happiness dwindles."

"Andrew, hold still. This might hurt a little," I said. I began to remove the tape from the white gauze bandage on his leg.

"People will divorce their wives, change jobs, or work a hundred hours a week in desperation to buy things they believe will make them happy. They will self-medicate with alcohol or drugs—anything to take away the pain. You know what? It never works. People try to change others or buy things to fill voids in their life. You can't fill a human need such as happiness with an object," he said. "I understand now that happiness needs to come from within."

I looked at his incision site. It had pink edges of healthy tissue and silver staples perfectly spaced apart. He was healing well. I replaced the bandage.

He paused and looked up at me. He placed his hand upon my forearm to make sure I was listening. "True happiness only occurs with a deep spiritual connection with a power greater than us. And I believe that connection is already present within each of us. We just need to find a way to turn it on."

I nodded my head in agreement, trying to comprehend exactly what he meant.

"Do you mind if I look at it?" I asked.

"No, of course not," he said.

He handed me the book, and I sat down beside him, thumbing through it. On the front cover was a picture of the Dalai Lama, the spiritual leader of Tibet, a man of peace and love. He was draped in burgundy and saffron holy robes. His balding head was in plain view, and his rectangular glasses were not quite perfect for his face. His smile was sweet, his eyes gentle and reassuring.

Something told me that he was not concerned about the way his glasses looked on him. He was more interested in spirituality and the human existence—people loving one another, taking care of those less fortunate, worshipping, and serving. He would leave the rest of the nonsense up to the world around him, the people who were caught up in the daily grind of life. At times, I've looked at myself in the mirror, and I've seen that person who is caught up in life. I don't like what I see in those moments.

When I left Andrew's room, I ventured back out into the world, and I tried to incorporate the principles that Andrew taught me. And now, when I drift off track, I think about the great lesson I learned from him.

We are all searching for happiness, but we'll never find it externally. It must come from within. It's a feeling I want to carry with me wherever I go.

∾

A WEEK PRIOR TO MEETING ANDREW, IN THE SPRING OF 1998, I had scribbled in my journal: "the machine of life has many moving parts." A random thought that struck me while sitting on a bench just before entering the hospital. That morning, I'd felt a general sense of uneasiness—the type of feeling that something in my life was wrong, but I couldn't quite put my finger on it. I wrote the phrase not knowing exactly why or what I even meant by it. I hoped that eventually the thought would settle in and make sense.

The day I met Andrew, I'd woken up without any precon-ceived notion of what the day would bring. I took life at face value. I simply lived in the present. That night, as I put my head on the pillow, I thought about how much richer my life had become.

Just as there are those days when nothing seems to go right, there are days when everything seems to fall in line. You leave with an unsuspected surprise—a day that warms your heart and calms your soul. This was one of those days.

Andrew gave me the answer I had been searching for. The parts of our lives—our intimate relationships, friendships, careers, hopes and dreams, aspirations, fears, our weaknesses and strengths—each part plays a role. Sometimes the machine hums along without any intervention. Occasionally it requires maintenance. We must address the problems that surface in our life. Blame doesn't fix them. And they don't go away by self-medication or ignoring them. They just compound like a wet snowball rolling down a hill. And the snowball becomes big enough to run over anything in its way.

Our first reaction is to try to temporarily fix things. We rush to try to make substitutions. Sometimes we end our friendships, change careers, sabotage relationships, give up on our hopes and dreams, succumb to our weaknesses. We look at the world around us and try to change it all in the desperate attempt to find happiness. But we never really address the true reason that we are unhappy.

What motivates us? I believe Andrew was right—it's happiness. But in order to find it, we must first look in the right place. And that place resides soundly within the center of your being. You won't find it in trying to change the world around you. In order to fix something, you must first know where to look. The machine of life is located inside us. And when we find true happiness, the moving parts of life work beautifully together, with little effort and in perfect harmony. They are each notes in a beautiful symphony, and they silently fall into their place.

Awakening from Near Death

Although my near-death experience was nearly thirty-four
years ago, there is virtually not a day that goes by that
I am not aware of making decisions based on that experience.

—GERALDINE BERKHEIMER

It's a balmy spring in 1976, and I am well into my seventh year on
this earth. My mother is a registered nurse working the evening
shift at a hospital in Cherry Hill, New Jersey. I awake to the
sound of her crying when she returns home from the hospital.
I walk downstairs and ask her, "Why are you crying?" I recall
wanting to cry too.

"I'll explain it to you when you get older," she says. "Later,
you'll understand."

"When?" I ask.

"How about when you turn nine?" And with that she turns
out my light and kisses me on the forehead.

Although I've thought of it often, I don't mention it again
until my ninth birthday. Just before bed, I ask her about that
night. "You promised," I remind her.

She steps back in amazement. It takes her a moment to collect her thoughts but she is able to remember every detail of our conversation. She sits beside me on my bed and speaks in a soft voice.

"That night a man that I was caring for died. His heart stopped beating. We called the doctors. They rushed into the room and brought him back to life. After the doctors left, I was left alone with the patient. And when he awoke he was angry, and he took it out on me."

She sees I don't understand by the bewildered look on my face.

"He asked me, 'How could you do that to me? I was in the most beautiful place, and all my pain was gone. Why did you have to get involved?'

"I was upset and confused. I thought we were doing the right thing. But now I understand why he was upset."

"I don't understand," I said. "You helped save his life."

"Yes—but we were the ones who didn't want to let go—not him."

Summer of 1998

Second Year of Medical Residency

I FOUND IT INTERESTING THAT WHEN LOUDEN'S FAMILY AND friends described him, they always referred to his heart. "Such a kindhearted man . . . full of heart . . . heart of gold," they would say.

Louden had a good heart when it came to the things that really mattered in life. He was a good friend, a caring son, and a faithful husband and father. But as an organ, his heart failed him early in life. At the age of forty-two he suffered his first heart attack.

I met Louden after he was recovering from cardiac bypass surgery. The surgery had taken a lot out of him, and he needed rehabilitation to regain his strength. A large white bandage spread across his chest. He was weak and his skin pale. Small beads of sweat glistened from his forehead. He breathed in oxygen from a clear tube that projected from the wall.

"Did they tell you what happened to me?" He quietly cleared his throat.

"Yes, I know about your surgery," I said as I handed him a tissue.

"No . . ." He looked at me for a moment with a puzzled look. "Did they tell you about the near-death experience?"

"No, I hadn't heard."

"Really?" He seemed disappointed. "They didn't tell you? I mean, I told my surgeon all about it. I thought for sure he would tell you."

I shook my head.

He rolled his eyes and took in a deep, long breath.

I often heard of the near-death experience and found it fascinating. It occasionally comes up in the hospital: on rounds, in the emergency room, when talking to family members of those who have almost died. It's one of those topics every doctor hears about, but on which no one is ready to take a stand— everyone is still sitting on the fence.

"Now you have to tell me," I said. "You can't just leave it at that."

He paused for a moment, deciding if he wanted to proceed. I could see the wheels of his mind turning until he couldn't hold back any longer. "Well, it all started while I was playing softball. I always promised myself this would be my last season. It was the second inning, and the pitcher threw one right over the plate. I ran as fast as I could. But as I rounded second base, my chest started squeezing and I couldn't breathe. I couldn't even make it to third base. The next thing I know there's an ambulance and I'm in the emergency room. They tell me I've had a heart attack."

I sat down beside him.

"That night they put a tube in my groin and injected some dye. They tell me I have a blockage in three of my vessels. The next morning I'm on the operating table. It all happened so fast."

"Thank God they found it," I said.

"Yes, but during the surgery there was a complication. I awoke and began to feel a sense of warmth. I could see a light—and then my spirit was hovering above the operating table."

He looked at me and sensed my disbelief. He held up his index finger with the rest of his hand in a fist. He shook his finger from side to side.

"Hold on now—just listen. It will make sense," he said. "So, as I'm floating there, looking down on my body, I see the anesthesiologist pushing medications into my arm. 'It's not working' he said. I see a flat line on a screen where your heart is supposed to be beating. I see my heart surgeon walk up to my chest and start massaging my heart. Suddenly, my spirit above the table disappears."

I was still hesitant to believe, but continued to listen.

"So I wake up in the post-op area hours later. I see my surgeon standing at the nurse's station talking to a nurse. He sees that I'm awake and walks in. The first thing I said to him was, 'Thank you for massaging my heart.' He looked at me, confused, and looked around the room. It was clear he was nervous and uncomfortable."

"What did the surgeon say?" I asked.

"He looked at me, and the first words out of his mouth were, 'Who told you about that?' I told him I hadn't talked to anyone—I saw it happen. He gave me some story about how hallucinations are common after surgery. Maybe it was due to anesthesia or possibly a dream. I told him directly to his face, 'It was as real as you and me sitting here talking right now.' He told me I was tired and I needed to sleep. Have you ever heard of such a thing?" Louden asked me.

I nodded. "I have before—it occurs occasionally. We just don't know how to explain it."

"Well, neither do I. But I want you to know what I saw was real. It was real." He laid his head back farther into the pillow. The white pillow wrapped around his head, almost covering his ears. He breathed in through his mouth and exhaled long and slowly.

"I don't have a great answer, either—but how can you explain millions of people—all across the world, with different religions and cultures and languages, who have never met—all sharing a similar story in their brief time between this world and their afterlife?" he asked.

A fair and excellent question with which the greatest minds in medicine have struggled, tried to resolve, but still to this day can't answer.

As I stood at his doorway, he left me with one final thought. He spoke in a measured tone, as if a metronome were playing in his mind, pacing the flow of his words and thoughts. "Believe it or not, the hardest part of this whole thing wasn't the surgery itself; it's what happened after. I didn't need my surgeon to confirm my experience; what I felt was real. I know that—all I needed was for him to listen to me, and he didn't. That hurt far more than being cut."

Some people can mend your heart and break it at the same time. I've seen it time and time again.

∾

AS A YOUNG CHILD, I WISHED I KNEW EVERYTHING. I CAN remember being six years old and tossing a penny into a fountain on a Sunday morning after church. As the water rippled, I made my wish to know everything in the world. It never came true, and I am so glad it didn't. The older I get, the more I appreciate the things I don't know. Not knowing everything keeps my eyes and ears open to the world around me. In this mind-set, life is more interesting. I remain fascinated with human anatomy and physiology. I love the complexity of human psychology. I also enjoy looking at controversial topics with open eyes to try to gain a better understanding.

When I think about some of the greatest medical discoveries, I can assure you that when they occurred, there was always a fair share of nonbelievers in the crowd. Those discoverers were willing to be ridiculed for their courage to think outside the box. Those willing to take risks, even if they look foolish, often end up making the greatest discoveries.

Louden didn't expect his surgeon to agree with him, nor did he expect his surgeon to have all the answers. He wanted to share with his surgeon his experience in the hope that he would listen and understand. His feelings were hurt because his surgeon didn't listen.

Recently I was asked again my feelings about the near-death experience. Do I believe it? Is it real? The truth is, I don't know—I'm still sitting on the fence. But now I sit there with open ears and an inquisitive mind.

And as I sit on the fence, gravity is leaning me toward believing.

In Search of Faith

Being religious means asking passionately
the question of the meaning of our
existence and being willing to receive
answers even if the answers hurt.

—Paul Tillich

*It's just shy of five o'clock in the morning as we begin surgery
rounds in the fall of 1994—my third year of medical school. The
sun waits patiently to light the sky. I have left the classroom of
medical school, and now I am in the hospital, taking care of real,
live patients. We sift through the final checklist to begin a long day
of surgery. We stand outside the main door of the operating room
next to a red line of tape on the floor. When that line is crossed,
the door automatically opens.*

*"Did you get the consents signed?" the attending surgeon
asks a fellow medical student.*

*"I did. Just one problem—the woman in room 305. Well,
she's a Jehovah's Witness. And if there is a complication, she has
refused a blood transfusion."*

"And what do you think about that?" the attending surgeon asks the student.

"Obviously, I don't think it's smart. She has dramatically increased her risk of dying on the table." He smiles and looks around at the other medical students, hoping for nods of approval.

The attending physician walks close to the student and crosses his boundaries of personal space. The medical student stiffens.

"As physicians, we do not let our personal beliefs influence the care of the patient. Do you understand me?"

The medical student nods.

"You are here to serve your patients, not judge them. I don't care what religion they are. You must always respect their wishes—always."

And with that, the surgeon walks across the red line on the floor. The entrance doors of the operating room swing open, and we all follow him in.

Fall of 1998

Third Year of Medical Residency

I KNOCKED ON JOY'S DOOR EARLY IN THE MORNING. THE HOSpital was quiet, the first peaceful moments before a storm was to blow in. I gave the door two swift knocks, then leaned my head around it.

"May I come in?" I asked.

"Sure, Doctor, come on in," she said.

Joy sat beside her bed in a reclining chair. She was crocheting—effortlessly pulling and tugging at the baby-blue thread, making knitted loops with a crochet hook.

"What are you making, Joy?" I asked.

"A baby blanket for my grandson. My baby girl just had a baby boy," she said, grinning from ear to ear.

I sat beside her and watched as she continued, stitch by stitch, to build a blanket out of thread. Occasionally she would look down, but her hands worked without having to see. She felt the needle in her hand—every stitch seemed effortless.

Her eyes were fixated on the television up in the corner of the room.

Joy was in her late sixties. She had a soft reassuring voice, dark beautiful skin, and a calm presence. She had been born and raised in a rural town in Alabama—a farming town with crops and cotton fields—plenty of hard work to go around. She grew up in a small home on five acres, and each inch of land was used to grow something for the family to eat. Eleven children were a lot of mouths to feed. What they didn't eat, they tried to sell. There were cows to milk, corn to shuck, and cotton to pick—each child lent a helping hand.

In the town center had been a grocery store, a post office, and a church where everyone gathered once a week. In good times and bad, they congregated each Sunday to find guidance in the teachings of the Bible and in one another's company. The church had made them a community.

When I think of church, I think of rows of families sitting in pews, listening to the preacher speak. Joy's church hadn't been like that—it was a gospel church. "We would sing and dance. We wore our finest clothes. We left energized, ready to face the world and the challenges of the week ahead."

Joy was in the hospital because her heart was failing her, and her blood pressure became more difficult to control. We were able to make her heart pump more effectively so fluid no longer built up in her lungs, but her blood pressure would suddenly rise to a dangerous level. We were concerned she would have a stroke. The nurse informed me that her hypertension had worsened.

"I hear your blood pressure is up. I just need to make sure we don't need to change your medication," I said.

She turned to me. "You look tired. You didn't get a wink of sleep, did you?"

"It was busy last night, Joy," I said.

"Why don't you go get some sleep and come back and check on me later? I ain't going anywhere," she said.

"I'm fine, Joy," I said. "But thank you."

Her dietician arrived and brought her breakfast: bacon, grits, and eggs. We had placed her on a strict diet; it was clear the dietician had brought her the wrong plate. She looked up at me and placed one finger in the middle of her lips as if to say, "Shhh." The dietician left.

"You aren't going to take this away from me, are you?" she asked.

"Just the bacon," I replied. I took a small packet of salt off her plate. "And no salt."

She interlocked her fingers and bowed her head in prayer. "Thank you, oh heavenly Father, for this wonderful meal, for the strength to carry on, for my family, my friends, and your ever-enduring love." She shot a wink at me. "And thank you for my doctor. In your name I pray. Amen."

I pumped up a blood pressure cuff on her arm and placed a stethoscope against her skin to listen. Her blood pressure was elevated.

"We're going to have to increase your blood pressure medication," I said.

She was looking over my shoulder as I told her this.

"Joy, did you hear me?" I asked.

"Yes. I'll tell you why my blood pressure is high." She points to the television, and CNN is rolling one tragic news story after another. A suicide bomber in the Middle East killed innocent tourists, a priest in New York City confessed to molesting a child, and an arsonist in Tennessee is charged with burning down a church.

"God must be looking down on us from above and shaking his head, wondering how we got so far off the path," she said.

"It's been a rough week on the news," I replied.

"It's a lot more than that, Doctor," she said.

I knew where this conversation was headed—religion. It was something I never felt comfortable talking about with patients, but it came up often. There has always been an intimate relationship between medicine and faith. Hand in hand they have walked together, like old friends. With illness and pain come thoughts of mortality, and we look for a higher power to heal us.

When asked about my personal beliefs, I would quickly change the subject. But with Joy I felt comfortable—not threatened—and I needed some guidance.

Lately, my faith had been shaken. I questioned my trust in a higher power. It wasn't one event that had left my spiritual tank empty; it was a few tragic events close together.

While moonlighting in the emergency room, I had performed an examination on a young woman who had been raped by three men at a local college. Her trusted boyfriend had escorted her to a party, and he and his two best friends had taken advantage of her. I had to examine her to record the evidence of the assault. The last thing in the world she'd wanted was to be touched by another man.

A few days later, I'd taken care of an eight-year-old boy whose father had beaten him with a metal shovel and burned him with cigarettes. I'd surveyed his bruises and burnt flesh. I'd looked into his empty, hollow eyes and tried to explain that people did love him. I knew he didn't believe me—I didn't blame him.

I thought, if there is a God, then how does He let this happen?

"Your faith, Joy—it's that important to you?" I asked.

"My belief in God is more important to me than any physical part of me. It's the foundation for how I live my life. I can tell you this—we are far off track. I don't care if you're a Christian, Buddhist, Jewish, Islamic, or Hindu—killing, lying, cheating, and deceiving in the name of religious beliefs are wrong. It's supposed to be about the love of your creator, having mercy, taking care of those less fortunate, and loving one another. How in the world did we get so far off track?"

She then turned her head away from the television and went back to her meal.

Joy was not the most articulate or educated woman I've ever met, but I will tell you this—she lived her life on a far better plane than most people with advanced degrees. She understood living, and she helped me regain my faith. Her method of teaching was simple—she didn't lecture; she taught by example. All I had to do was watch.

I turned to the window and watched the storm blow in, and smiled as the rain fell.

∾

MY INTEREST IN SPIRITUALITY AND RELIGION CAME TO ME later in life. It began after my meeting Joy, as we entered into a new millennium. And the world around me lived in fear of the unknown. The media fueled the fire and then capitalized on the very fear it created. Some people sold their belongings and withdrew their money from their banks, and the sale of generators went through the roof. Some of the headlines read: "The End Is Near."

But for some reason I never bought into the hype. I wasn't as afraid of the unknown. My interest lay in finding a common thread that weaved its way throughout the religions of the world.

It began from an interest in the relationship between medicine and healing. It evolved into a personal journey. Perhaps, like many of you, I was looking to make sense of the world around me, a process of introspection that began one day when

I vowed to ask myself the all-important question—if I were to die today, what would happen to me? And followed with the question: Is this all there is to life? It evolved, for me, into the idea that there must be something more.

As physicians, we are called upon to treat people of all religions and denominations. What is it that ties each of us together regardless of which God we choose to worship? The thought crossed my mind that maybe it was more of a principle. I thought that maybe the Golden Rule—do unto others as you would have others do unto you—seemed to fit perfectly into this belief. The belief in an afterlife smoothed out the top, and hope and faith rounded out the edges. Maybe we all have more in common than we imagined.

When I met Joy, I had more questions than answers. I wondered if there was a common thread at all. How can people do such heinous acts in the name of religion? She taught me that people often do a poor job of representing the higher power they choose to worship. They taint religion with their own man-made ideology and attribute it to God. Religious extremism—as with any beliefs taken to an extreme—will often end in destruction, even if those beliefs begin with the best of intentions. Religion's greatest challenge lies in man's interpretation of religion—especially when used to manipulate others for personal gain.

But most importantly, Joy revealed to me the answer I was searching for. She taught me that the common thread of all religions is love. And I believe that God is love.

First Do No Harm

Declare the past, diagnose the present, foretell the
future; practice these acts. As to diseases, make a habit
of two things—to help, or at least do no harm.

—Hippocrates, *Epidemics*

*I'm twelve years old in the summer of 1981 and flipping through
magazines next to my father's chair. I come across an article about
a young doctor who took his own life.*

*He was a young pediatrician from a small Southern town
who was treating a child for strep throat. He peeked in with a
light and saw the classic signs: the white patches on the corners
of his tonsils, the red and angry throat. He decided to give the
child a shot of penicillin as he had thousands of times before.*

*As soon as he did, the child became limp and grabbed at his
throat. His skin turned blue and then ashen. The mother, a dear
friend of his family, started screaming. The doctor injected him
with adrenaline and tried to maintain his airway. They performed CPR, but the child died in front of him and the boy's
mother.*

The doctor was devastated. He canceled his afternoon, got into his car, and drove home to see his wife and children. And as his wife and children waited for him on the porch at home, the doctor pulled his car over to the side of the road. He reached into his glove compartment for his gun, which was always there for safety. He now meant it to serve a different purpose. He angled the barrel of the gun against his temple, and pulled the trigger.

For all these years, this story has remained in the back of my mind. When I think about the young child and his mother and the pain he must have suffered, I understand why he felt he couldn't go on.

Being a physician is a great responsibility, and not something to be taken lightly. I treasure that responsibility.

I'm not here to pass judgment on the way he chose to handle his grief. I simply pray that if I'm ever in a similar situation, I will have the strength to handle myself differently. It's only in the past five years that I've come to believe I would have the strength to carry on. His story resonated with me for a reason.

Winter of 1999

Third Year of Medical Residency

"WE MUST DO SOMETHING," THE NURSE SAID TO ME AS SHE rubbed Joan's shoulders.

Joan sat slumped in a wheelchair with a pink shawl draped around her neck. Her face was wrinkled and void of expression. From the corner of her mouth, saliva would drool and trickle off her chin. The nurse placed an emesis basin in her lap with a towel to catch her secretions. Joan would stare at an object for minutes, then she would find a new object and begin the process again. She was present but not mentally aware. Her mind was tangled with cobwebs.

When people saw her they whispered, "Dementia," or "Poor thing, isn't Alzheimer's terrible?" I wasn't convinced she had either one. She looked tired, in a trance, and disconnected from the world.

I was new to the rehabilitation rotation. When the physicians were deciding which patients we would follow, I mentioned that I would like to take care of her.

"Good luck—she just arrived last week. Be sure you keep her daughters informed of all medication changes. It will serve you well in the long run," the attending said.

I nodded and didn't say a word.

After rounds that morning I went to talk to her daughters. Both were in their early fifties. One daughter had sandy blond hair and an introverted personality. Her sister was brunette and extroverted.

"I can't believe that no one can do anything with my mother. You have to understand that we are very frustrated. We have been to so many doctors, and no one, I mean no one, has done anything for her," the brunette sister said.

"Who have you seen?" I asked.

"Well, we took her to our family practice doctor because our mother was forgetful and having trouble sleeping. He put her on a memory pill and a sleeping pill. She was still having trouble during the day, so he sent her to a neurologist. He did an MRI of her brain and drew some blood. Everything was all right. He gave her something different to help her sleep, and to calm her nerves during the day."

Her sister interrupted. "And don't forget the psychiatrist."

The extroverted sister continued. "Well, she seemed depressed, so we took her to a psychiatrist. He placed her on an antidepressant. Two weeks later, we revisited him. She still seemed depressed, so he gave her something else to try. She then became even more agitated and difficult to take care of. He then gave her something to calm her down. She keeps getting worse."

She pointed across the room at her mother.

"She was working in her garden two months ago. Now she's sitting in the corner drooling, unable to stand or walk, and every test we get back is negative. Nobody can find anything wrong with her. Please help us," she said.

That night on the way home, I was thinking about Joan. Nothing quite made sense. In the early stages of Alzheimer's, patients don't become detached and lose contact with the world so rapidly. There was no significant change on the MRI of her brain. Her labs were essentially normal. Nothing was adding up.

And then it hit me—I wondered if the daughters were giving her every pill that each doctor along the way had prescribed.

I came to work early the next morning before the medications were dispensed. I asked the nurse, "Who is giving Joan her medications?"

"Her daughters. They refused to let us give her medication."

I went into the room and talked to both daughters. "I think I know what's wrong with your mom. Would you mind showing me her medications?"

"Of course not," the outgoing one said. They pulled out two bags of prescription medicine.

"Now, which ones are you giving her every day?"

"All of them," she replied.

I sorted through the medications. Joan was on sleeping pills, two antidepressants, two medicines for anxiety, a muscle relaxer, a narcotic for pain, and an Alzheimer's medication—not including other pills for her heart failure and blood pressure.

I told the daughter, "I think I know why she's like she is. It's called polypharmacy. She is on entirely too much medication."

"But her doctors put her on these for a reason. Why would they have done that?"

I asked her if she had told the doctors about prior doctor visits and the medications her mother was on. "No, I assumed they knew."

They didn't. They had been embarrassed to tell each new doctor whom they had seen previously. They didn't want to seem like they were doctor shopping. More was better in their minds. The doctors were trying to help Joan and so were her daughters. It was a breakdown of communication—too many people trying to do the right thing.

Over the next week I tapered her off all of her medications except for her blood pressure medications, her heart failure medication, and her memory medication. Each and every day she improved. The cobwebs cleared from her mind. She began listening to music, even sitting in her chair and swaying with a sense of rhythm. She talked again.

I learned a myriad of lessons from Joan. All have served me well in my life spent in medicine. Above all, first do no harm. Don't ever underestimate the power of communicating with everyone involved in a patient's care. Don't ever assume. Think logically and clearly before intervening with the body's natural state and prescribing medication. Sometimes we try so hard to help others that our good intentions get in the way of the end result. Sometimes a guarded approach works best, with a cautious and watchful eye and a belief in the human body to heal. The body has a tremendous capacity to heal—sometimes we just need the discipline to let it.

∾

SOMETIMES SEEING THE SMALLEST RESULTS IN A PATIENT CAN reap great rewards. Seeing Joan's mind clearing of cobwebs and her ability to function again was a special moment for me. With a few adjustments, the quality of her life improved tremendously. I took great pride in watching her improve daily. The last day, she stood up, walked out of her wheelchair, and hugged me. At that moment, her daughters knew they had their mother back.

I went over this case in my mind many times to be sure that nothing similar would happen again. It instilled in me the importance of taking a meticulous history. There is a great danger in a doctor practicing medicine based on false assumptions. I consistently remind myself never to assume.

We physicians are blessed to have a variety of tools to heal at our disposal, but often our tools are best left in the toolbox. Medications can sometimes serve our patients better in the bottle than flowing through their bloodstream.

Stopping Your World
for a Friend

A real friend is one who walks in
when the rest of the world walks out.

—WALTER WINCHELL

We hand in our final exams of our third year of medical school in the late spring of 1995. A group of fellow students quickly heads to the local tavern. We try to remember as many questions as we can and compare answers. When the tavern closes, we head to a friend's house. We pull out some lawn chairs and stare at the stars. With a cocktail in one hand and a celebratory cigar in the other, we toss around ideas of what to do with our newfound freedom of summer. We find great pleasure in doing the very things we know we shouldn't be doing. The world feels wide open.

"How about we go to the beach?"

"Too hot."

"How about we go up north?"

"No . . . humidity is still there."

"How about we go across country? Let's go out west."

We all look at one another and nod our heads. "Perfect," we say. And we all promise that no matter what, we will take the trip together.

A week before the trip my future wife asks me to stay. "Stay here with me," she says. "Please don't go."

I decided to stay. I was in love, and I chose her over them. It was a difficult decision. My friends were disappointed and gave me grief. But they laughed it off in time. And then they left without me.

While in Nevada, my friends were involved in a car accident. One friend was killed. My other friends were injured. It was blind luck that I wasn't there. But you don't feel lucky when a friend dies. My friend was smart and charismatic, and would have made an excellent physician. He was one of the smartest people I've ever met. I miss him. And I can't help but wonder if the accident would have happened if I'd gone with them. A part of me wishes I had. Maybe things would have been different. Maybe I would have been driving. Maybe I could have prevented it. Maybe Michael would still be alive.

Maybe . . .

Spring of 1999

Third Year of Medical Residency

T OM AWOKE IN A HOSPITAL ROOM AND TRIED TO MAKE SENSE of his surroundings. His vision was blurry, and his eyelids were heavy. The narcotics clouded his mind.

He heard a voice. "Tom ... it's Mick. You've been in an accident. I'm here—everything is fine. Go back to sleep."

Tom closed his eyes and smiled, knowing his best friend was beside him.

On a spring day in Atlanta, the day after Tom turned twenty-three, his car was hit as he made his way through an intersection. He didn't see it coming, and the man who hit him plowed right into his door. Tom lay in his car, unable to move, surrounded by shattered glass. As he lay there, all he could think about was his wife and Mick. His best friend, Mick, had always been there to protect him, and now he wasn't. He felt alone.

When his wife arrived at the hospital, some of the first words out of Tom's mouth were, "Call Mick. He would want to know."

In Boston, when Mick heard the news, he said to Tom's wife, "I'll be right there."

He flew to Atlanta that night and remained with Tom until he recovered. He stayed by his bedside night and day. He helped Tom's wife take care of their children. He went to get them food when they were hungry. He rocked them to sleep. He kept track of Tom's medicines to make sure there were no errors in judgment.

One morning I saw Mick in the hospital cafeteria.

"Do you mind if I take a seat?" I asked.

"Please, help yourself," he said. He was staring at the bacon and eggs on his plate. His mind seemed in another place.

"Mick, you have been real good to Tom. Everyone needs a friend like you," I said.

He looked at me. "That's what friends are for. I did exactly for him what he would have done for me. You would have done the same thing."

I nodded my head, but wondered deep down inside if it was true. Would I have stopped my world to take care of a friend? It was a phase in my life when I was not a good friend. The time commitment of medicine had taken its toll. I did not rise to the occasion. There were calls I did not return. There were weddings I missed. There were times when my friends needed me, and I was not there for them.

"What did your boss say about you leaving?" I asked.

"Well, I'm sure he's not happy, but he'll have to get over it."

"And your wife—does she understand?" I asked.

"She doesn't understand it completely, but she'll forgive me. She met Tom after college, so she never really knew how close we were. I don't know if this makes sense, but it would be easier to ask for forgiveness from them than to try to forgive myself."

"You guys are that close?" I asked.

"Tom is like my brother. He's closer to me than many people in my family. We've been friends since we were eight.

We went to the same school, played street hockey every afternoon, and had our first kiss with the same girl. Even though we were the same age, he was like a little brother to me. A friendship like that doesn't end just because you grow older or your lives take a different path. There will always be a bond between us—always."

In Mick I saw a younger version of myself, but more idealistic, more compassionate. The educational process and the daily grind of life had extinguished that part of me. I wanted to rekindle it.

The morning of Tom's discharge from the hospital, I saw him hobble out of the elevator on crutches. His wife was on one side and Mick on the other. They walked out through automatic doors into the bright yellow sun. I stood and watched, as Mick opened the door for Tom, how Tom reached his arm around Mick's neck and how he gently slid him into the seat. Mick closed the car door behind him and climbed into the back of the car. I watched them drive off together.

At that moment, I made myself a promise—I would become a better friend. No matter what, I would become a better friend.

∾

I'M BLESSED TO HAVE AN ECLECTIC GROUP OF FRIENDS THAT remain such an important part of my life. Our lives have led us in many directions, but we're still the same in so many ways. We're sobered by responsibility. The world no longer revolves around us.

During the time I took care of Tom, I struggled to find a balance between the demands of career and my commitment to being a good friend. Friendship is not bound by blood or legality; you can walk away at any time. But based on our love for another, we choose to stay. It is a relationship that is honest in intention and simplistic in its foundation. Although I was not there for them, my friends stayed.

As we progress through life, the role of friendship in our lives changes. It no longer remains the cornerstone of our existence as it does in our developmental years and through early adult life. It takes a backseat to building a family. When we begin a family, we are confronted with new demands and new responsibilities. Good friends understand this.

I once thought the true test of a friendship was the willingness to drop everything to take care of a friend. But now I realize it's more than that. A good friend stays with you whether you're in their physical presence or not.

They're there within you always... no matter what.

Watching People Fall

There are all kinds of addicts, I guess.
We all have pain. And we all look for ways
to make the pain go away.

—SHERMAN ALEXIE,
THE ABSOLUTE TRUE DIARY OF A PART-TIME INDIAN

It's my first night in the emergency room as a medical intern in the summer of 1997. My first of four years of medical residency are beginning, and I'm looking for ways to survive.

The medical residents stand at the nurses' station while the attending physician talks to the charge nurse. Just before rounds, a fellow resident nudges me with his elbow. He has two more years of experience under his belt and feels he has figured out the room before we begin. We have a few moments to kill, and he decides to play a game. My mind is wide open to new ideas.

"You see that guy over there?" he asks. He turns his head toward me; his voice is just above a whisper. He points to a skeleton of a man who lies in a bed flat on his back with a sheet only half-covering his body. "Methamphetamines."

"How can you tell?" I ask.

"You can always tell by the hollow cheeks and the rotten teeth."

He points to a homeless man in the corner. "That guy is a drinker. You can always tell the veteran drunks versus the binge drinkers."

"How?"

"It's July and hot as hell outside. He's wearing gloves and a jacket. The binge drinkers are fat. The hard-core alcoholics—the ones that drink hard liquor—they eventually quit eating. So when they choose between liquor and food, they're always going to choose liquor. So they don't have any body fat to keep them warm."

He senses that I'm impressed. "Don't worry. It will come. You'll be able to do it too. Unfortunately, the downside is you'll never be able to look at the world the same way again."

Fall of 1999

Fourth Year of Medical Residency

I SAT DOWN AND WATCHED THE EVENING NEWS BEFORE leaving for my night shift in the emergency room. During residency, I moonlighted in the emergency room to pay off medical school debt. Every day the debt clock ticked, and it was never in my favor.

I was running late and glanced frequently at my watch. I tried to steal a few more moments.

The anchorman sat with his forearms resting comfortably on the long desk in front of him. He sat upright, his fingers interlaced. The large window behind him framed the lights and skyscrapers of New York City. He looked immaculate: his hair neatly combed, a pinstripe suit, his faced neatly powdered. He stared directly into the camera.

He spoke with a deep calm voice. "Ladies and gentleman, I have some good news for you—America is winning the war on drugs." He smiled.

This is wonderful, I thought. I grabbed my white coat and headed out the door.

As I walked down the center of the aisle in the emergency room, I noticed it was unusually crowded. The halls were lined with stretchers; there weren't enough rooms for the wounded. I began my shift in the Red Zone—red stands for blood, and that night there was plenty.

I stopped for a moment and took it all in as a simple thought floated through my mind. The emergency room was filled with people in various shades of gray regarding mental clarity and psychological stability. There were those who were there because their behavior had hurt them, and there were those who had been hurt by the behavior and actions of others. Life found a way for them to be at the wrong place at the wrong time. Any given night is unpredictable at best. A doctor must always be alert and ready to react.

Off to my left lay a middle-aged man with a gunshot wound to his left leg. As I approached him, the smells of hard liquor, urine, and body odor filled my nose. His head nodded rhythmically in almost slow motion. A white bandage, wrapped tightly around his leg, had turned red and seeped with blood.

I continued toward the nursing station, and I saw a teenager handcuffed to his stretcher. He wore a ripped blue T-shirt and baggy jeans. He had a gauze bandage wrapped tightly around his head, and a bag of ice rested against his cheek. Every once in a while he pulled the handcuff against the stretcher just to see if it was really attached—even though he knew it was.

I stepped a few feet farther and saw a thirty-five-year-old woman lying in bed. She was crying after having been beaten. Her eyes were swollen and bruised; there was a cut across her cheek. She spit blood into an emesis basin.

I walked up to the nurses' station, and a resident eagerly awaited my arrival.

"Man, I am so glad to see you," he said. He looked young to be a doctor—the face of a boy. He was thin, in green scrubs, and had brown slicked-back hair.

"It's a full moon tonight. The ICU is full, there are no beds anywhere—we don't have anyplace to put these people."

As we moved from the nurses' station, I heard noise in the detention area, the place where people under arrest were stabilized medically before being transferred to jail.

The resident looked in the direction of the noise. "It's probably the guy on PCP. The last time, he took four cops on—this time it looks like they've sent in reinforcements," he said.

I saw a group of police officers running full speed down the hall with one hand on their nightsticks and one on their guns.

My fellow resident and I walked toward the man who had been shot in the leg. It had been a long night, and the resident's compassion was waning. "So this guy and his friend are sharing some liquor. His friend decided to take more than his fair share. So he decides to shoot him. Reasonable enough. Well, his friend didn't fancy being shot, so he shot him back. Eye for an eye, so to speak."

The man turned and pleaded his case to me. "What he did wasn't right."

I don't say a word—it's easy for tensions to escalate. I knew soon he would go back to sleep and wake up with his leg pounding more than ever, and I hoped it would sink in that he and his friend had almost died over a five-dollar bottle of liquor.

We walked toward the young man who had been involved in the car accident, but before we got too close the resident stopped. "The police officer just informed him that his friend was killed in the car he was driving. He failed to see the road turn left and continued right. There were no tire marks at the scene. My bet is he was too drunk to see it coming. Probably passed out at the wheel. He's sobering up but going to jail soon," he said.

And then we walked into the room of the woman who had been beaten by her boyfriend. Her clothes were covered with blood. Her face was black and blue, and her eyes were swollen shut.

"Her boyfriend beat her up again. He's a frequent flyer here too. You've probably seen him around. He's always up to something—fighting, selling drugs, prostitution. I saw him in here last week. She's stable physically. We'll let the psychiatrists deal with the mental issues."

"All right, I'll be right back," I said to her.

"Dr. Kelly, is that you?" she asked.

There I stood, looking at a woman whose face was so battered I didn't recognize her.

"Sarah?" I asked.

"Yes. Dr. Kelly, this time I am going to leave him—I promise," she said.

The last time I'd seen her, her cocaine-addicted boyfriend had beaten her up, and she had promised to leave him. Each time it got progressively worse.

"Do you need anything?" I asked.

"No, I'm all right," she said.

"I'll be right back."

My resident and I continued down the hall until we had discussed each patient. He left with a final comment—"Have fun"—and he slapped me on the back.

I changed the gunshot victim's bandage. "General surgery will be coming for you soon," I said.

I talked to the young man who'd been in the car accident. He was worried about his parents' reaction. He tried to explain what had happened. "I just lost control, that's all. I didn't mean to hurt anyone." Unfortunately, we couldn't bring his friend back, and his life would never be the same. The handcuffs remained firmly around his wrists.

I checked on Sarah. I wanted to tell her to get out of the relationship. I wanted to give her advice, but not all advice here was welcomed. I examined her and washed out her wounds.

"You know, he used to not hit. He used to treat me real well," she said. She tried to clear her throat and hold back her tears.

"If I could just get him off those drugs, he's really not a bad person."

"Have you seen yourself yet? Your face—have you seen it?" I asked.

"No."

"I think you should. You might feel differently."

I supported her by the arm and gently led her to the mirror above the sink. She lifted her own eyelid to see the damage he had done. "Oh my God," she said. "This one is definitely the worst. What do you think I should do?" she asked.

"Listen—every time I see you, it gets worse and worse. The first time he pushed you down the stairs and hurt your wrist. The next time he kicked you and broke your ribs. Now he's begun to hit in the face, and once a man does that to a woman, it only gets worse."

"How would you know?" she asked.

"I've seen it time and time again in the emergency room. History tends to repeat itself."

"I know," she said. "I know."

I never saw her again.

I stood in the middle of the emergency room; all I could think of was how alcohol or drugs played a starring role in every case I saw that evening.

When the night was finished and I was about to leave, I saw a police officer standing outside the detention area where all the commotion had happened earlier. He was tall, six foot four, with broad shoulders, and biceps the size of my thighs.

"What happened earlier down here?" I asked.

"What do you think?" He raised his arm and pointed his index finger and scanned the emergency room. "Drugs—it's always drugs, isn't it? I swear to you, I've been doing this for twenty-five years, and it gets worse every day."

I thought back to the newscaster that evening, as he'd sat in the comfort of his studio while the world went on around him. America is winning the war on drugs?

Yeah, right.

∾

MY TIME SPENT IN THE EMERGENCY ROOM WAS A LOVE-HATE relationship. I loved the adrenaline rush of the action, the ability to learn and do things that I wouldn't otherwise do. The learning curve was steep but filled with opportunity. I tried to take away as much from the experience as I could.

But there was also a side that made me question the world around me and see the darker side of humanity. I saw firsthand what drugs did to people. I saw how drugs changed relationships, and how addiction left families destroyed in its wake. I saw many people lose their battle with addiction. I watched them fight their demons and lose.

It also opened my eyes to the influence of media. The older I get, the harder it is to discern where the influence of the media begins and ends. I constantly remind myself to look at the world with open eyes. I also realize how important it is to nourish my mind with things that will enhance my life. Those things are rarely found on television. I try to expose my mind to the beauty of the world—music, literature, and art.

I remember my last shift in the emergency room as if it were yesterday. I took off my white coat, folded it across the front seat of my car, and drove my car past an ambulance that was headed toward the trauma bay. I smiled and felt relieved as I headed home. I also remember hoping I would never return.

But as with any love-hate relationship, the more time passed, the more I couldn't help but dream about what could have been. I still drive by the same emergency room on my way to work each morning, and sometimes I can't help but wonder what I'm missing.

Moving Forward

The weak can never forgive.
Forgiveness is the
attribute of the strong.

—MAHATMA GANDHI

I am a medical student in the fall of 1994 and new to the life of being in the hospital. I try to figure out how the process of hospital rounds works. They seem much more intense than I imagined. At lunch, I see a medical resident on my team sitting in the corner of the hospital cafeteria. His face is long, and he seems disheartened. That morning, the attending physician had lit into him about a patient. I go over to check on him.

"I'm sorry about earlier this morning," I say. "Don't take it personally. It's happened to everyone on the service."

"It's not about that," he says. "My wife and I are having trouble."

"What happened? Not enough time at home?"

"Maybe to begin with, but now it's much worse. I had an affair."

We look at each other and don't speak. The fifteen seconds of void in conversation seems like an eternity. I mumble out, "Do you love her? The girl?"

"No. I realize now that I was simply trading temporary pleasure for happiness. I was miserable. I reached out to this other woman to help me. But, the truth is, it was never about her. It was about me. Now I have to deal with the consequences."

"Is your wife willing to work it out?"

"Well, she said she would try to forgive me. So we can work it out for the kids' sake. She said she would try to learn to trust me again. But right now, I'm wondering if I can ever forgive myself."

Winter of 2000

Fourth Year of Medical Residency

I STOOD BESIDE MY PATIENT, JENNIFER, AND NOTICED THAT the intravenous antibiotics were not flowing properly into her hand. I adjusted a kink in the tube, and then turned my attention to the needle. With every adjustment of the needle, her calm demeanor was unchanged. It was painful, but Jennifer didn't flinch. She understood pain.

At twenty-three years old, she had been diagnosed with leukemia. Her immune system remained weak, and she was battling her most recent episode of pneumonia. As I adjusted the needle in her hand, I noticed a small beaded bracelet across her wrist. Across the bracelet were the letters H-O-P-E.

"My father is coming to see me tomorrow," she said.

She handed me a frameless picture. It was faded and the edges were frayed.

"I haven't seen him since I was seven." Her eyes shifted to her wrist, and she began to play with her bracelet. "One night my parents were fighting, and he left. He never even said good-bye. My mother wouldn't let me contact him. And he never tried—no cards, no letters, no presents."

As I reached out for the picture, I could see the first tear turn the corner of her eye. I handed her a tissue and diverted my attention to the picture: It was the day of her christening. She was a baby with a long white dress that flowed well beyond her feet. Her mother and father stood side by side, each with a hand under Jennifer, supporting her. Her father grinned from ear to ear.

"It was a long time ago, but I need to find out why he left me."

The next morning, I stood at the nurses' station reviewing a chart. I recognized her father the moment I saw him walk through the elevator doors. He was much older, with softer features than the man in the picture I had seen. He took off his hat and played with it nervously in his hands.

"She's been waiting for you," I said.

He smiled.

I showed him to her room, and I watched as he sat down beside her. And then I left.

When I returned to check on her later that evening, I stopped outside her room and looked in. Her father sat in the same chair. He now sat closer, and they were holding hands. They laughed and smiled.

After visiting hours were over, I stopped by her room. As I entered, she looked up at me.

"You know, what people say is true—there are always two sides to a story. I thought this whole time my father didn't care." The tears poured from her eyes and rolled off her cheeks. She took quick, shallow breaths, trying to regain her composure.

"When I was eight, I had a ballet recital. All the parents were there except for my father. As I looked out across the audience, I thought I saw him in the back against a doorway. After the performance, I looked for him but he was gone. In my heart, I always thought it was my father. Tonight, I asked him about it. He had been there. He described the situation in detail. He also described a number of things along the way that I didn't know about. As it turns out, he has been watching me from a distance this whole time."

I sat beside her and listened.

"This whole time he has never remarried. I thought for sure he had. He said it was too painful for him to consider going through it again. I thought it was just me hurting, but he was hurting too."

"Do you think you will ever be able to forgive him?" I asked.

"I know I'll try. I know that the pain of not having him in my life is worse than my desire to hate him," she said. "Cancer has changed my world. Things seem much clearer now. There's no excuse for what he did, but my desire to have family around me is stronger than ever. So, if that means swallowing my pride, then that's what I'll do. I know it won't be easy with my mom, but I need him back in my life. I need to know my father. I need to forgive."

As I sat beside her, I saw her more clearly than ever before. A young lady, burdened by a difficult life, and I watched in amazement as she rose above it all.

∾

JENNIFER TAUGHT ME THAT THE DECISIONS WE MAKE AS ADULTS do not stop with us. They affect everyone around us too. When adults decide to have a family, we have a great responsibility. It is a responsibility we must cultivate, protect, and nourish.

Over the next few weeks, her father came to visit daily. It started with short visits, and then he ended up spending most of his days with his daughter. At first, her mother and father would coordinate times to be sure they wouldn't run into each other. A deep emotional barrier remained between them. Then Jennifer found a way to "accidentally" make sure they did see each other. She wanted closure not only for herself but for them too. It seemed her illness narrowed the distance between them.

On my last day of taking care of Jennifer, she told me her parents were going out for coffee.

"Really?" I said. I was surprised. I assumed the curtain on their relationship had been closed forever.

She smiled. "I believe in their own way they still love each other. When things fell apart, neither of them reached out.

Stubbornness and pride settled in. Neither would budge. Now they're old enough to know they need companionship... they need a friend."

"Who knows what will happen?" I said.

"Well, they're both still single," she said. A mischievous smile spread across her face. "Crazier things have happened."

Jennifer's ability to forgive gave her the strength to reach deep within to put closure to a painful situation. The thought of her parents being together gave her hope. And when her body was failing her and every moment of life was a struggle, she found great comfort in that hope.

She fiddled with her bracelet. "Hope is what brings us all together," she said. She seemed more content with the wind at her back as life presented her with new possibilities.

"And when the world comes crashing around me, I think of the word *hope*. And that's what keeps me living," she said.

What Money Can't Buy

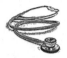

For any sensible person, money is two things:
a major liberating force, and a
great convenience. It's devastating to those
who have in mind nothing else.

—John Kenneth Galbraith

My four-year-old daughter stands next to me by the cash register at a local grocery store in the summer of 2006. The polite young cashier looks at my daughter and smiles as she passes our items across the scanner. When she finishes, my bags are full of groceries, and I hand her some money. My daughter watches with great interest as the cashier opens the cash register drawer and places the money in it. We go about our merry way.

On the way home, my daughter is quiet. I can tell her mind has wandered.

"What are you thinking about?" I ask.

"Well, if you hand people money, do they give you what you want?" she asks. She has just made one of life's little discoveries. I'm afraid it is too early and maybe not for the right reasons.

I nod.

"I want to be so rich, then."

Uh-oh, here we go. I can see her little mind working, and I tread forward with great trepidation. I know the many land mines that lurk around the corner. But I try to take advantage of the teachable moment.

"Yes, money does buy certain things . . . but it can't buy everything."

"How about candy or ice cream?"

"Yes."

"And dolls and princess costumes?"

"Yes. But it can't buy the most important things in life. Things like friendship, or love, or family."

And so for the next two weeks, each time my daughter brought up money, I made her repeat the things in life that were more important than money. Each time we asked her what she thought was more important than money, she would blurt out without hesitation, "Friendship, love, family."

I beamed with satisfaction, I was the proudest father on earth.

Fast forward, a month later. My wife and daughter sit in the kindergarten admissions office of a local school. My daughter seems calm and reserved. My wife, on the other hand, is trying her best to retain her composure. She is seasoned in the unpredictability of a four-year-old.

The interviewer begins with a simple question: "What's the most important thing to you?"

My wife is sitting next to her. She smiles knowing full well what's coming next—friendship, love, and family. She begins to breathe a sigh of relief.

My daughter pauses and cracks a mischievous smile. She looks directly at my wife and then at the interviewer. "Money."

Winter of 2000

Fourth Year of Medical Residency

M Y FAVORITE TIME TO VISIT JACK WAS IN THE EVENINGS. During the day, his hospital room became a stream of constant visitors. All visitors were colleagues from his law practice or former clients. His family was noticeably absent. There was a pile of unopened gifts left in the corner. The hours of visitation became a competition among those desperately searching for his attention.

Each visitor told a story about Jack's career in law. How he used the courtroom as a stage, and how he loved being the center of attention. He felt most comfortable with the light shining upon him and all eyes fixed in his direction. How he would do anything to capture the attention of the jury—standing on tables, raising his voice, and the relentless badgering of witnesses—a talent that had made him famous in local circles. And by the time the judge banged the final gavel down to call court to a close, Jack usually had won. In the process of perfecting his craft, Jack had made himself and his partners very wealthy.

I met Jack after he was diagnosed with pancreatic cancer. He had completed extensive surgery followed by radiation and chemotherapy. He was now in his mid-fifties, and his frame was thirty pounds lighter than at the peak of his career. The shock of the diagnosis, the thought of mortality, and the feeling of being alone had worn him down. His personal life was also in shambles. He faced an imminent divorce, and his children had alienated themselves from him. His colleagues talked of his toughness and his ruthlessness—I found him humane, respectful, and reserved.

I entered his room on a Wednesday evening. He had completed his dinner and was finishing his dessert. Earlier in the day, I had stopped by, but people from his office filled the room. He had politely asked me to come back later.

"I want to apologize to you," he said now.

"For what?" I asked.

"For earlier—for the circus in the room today. These people are used to being told what to do. Suddenly I can't tell them what to do—they're lost."

"I'm sure they mean well."

"Maybe, but you know there are other motives as well. That's why I find it hard to deal with it. Would you mind if I had no visitors tomorrow?"

"Of course not," I said.

"This whole cancer thing has really shaken me up a bit. I'm sorry." Tears welled up in his eyes; he paused and struggled to regain his composure.

I put down his chart on the bedside table, pulled up a chair, and sat next to him.

He paused and rested his head back against his pillow. "Being diagnosed with cancer is the strangest experience I've ever encountered. You spend your whole life trying to work hard to buy more things, and the second you get diagnosed—your desire to purchase is gone."

He sat up in his bed. "I have three homes but no one to share them with, a plane but no one to fly with me, and cars that I can't drive. Along the way I've destroyed my marriage and my relationship with my children, and the only people I really call friends are colleagues, not true friends. I have a lot of people around me, but I'm very alone. And all this, for what?"

He shook his head slowly from side to side. "I would trade it all for one more day with my wife and children."

I sat back and listened to him. I was a broke medical resident with mounting medical school debt, and the harder I worked, the more it grew. At times, I felt that I would never get ahead. I struggled just to keep my head above water.

I found myself envious of people with financial security. I admired their freedom. They could fly anywhere in the world without giving it a second thought. They spent their summers in their vacation homes and spent their winters skiing. I was guilty of assumption. I naively assumed their life was perfect.

"Have you talked to your family?" I asked.

"No, I don't even think they know I'm here. My wife and I separated quite some time ago."

"Well, Jack, there's never a better time than now. I think you should call them."

"Do you think so?"

"Absolutely."

The next morning Jack called his wife and his two children. He asked them to come see him. He told them how much he loved them and how sorry he was, and how cancer taught him what really mattered in his life.

As it turned out, they all showed up. The emotional walls that Jack had built around himself dissolved, and he was able to let his family back into his life. His children sat in his hospital room and helped him with the unopened presents stacked in the corner. He lived the remainder of his short life being the husband and father he had always wanted to be.

An experience, as Jack would say, "money could never buy."

∾

THE LAST EVENING I SPENT WITH JACK HE REMAINED IN GOOD spirits, but he was still trying to come to terms with how his life had taken a turn for the worse. His mind still churned, and his heart filled with regret about how his life had drifted off track. He pushed away the things that meant the most to him.

That evening he told me, "When life got challenging, I focused on my work. It was something I found great comfort in. I realized I was good at it. I felt that if I was providing for my family then they had no reason to question me as a father and a husband. I realize now I could have had it all."

Later, upon reading my notes on Jack, I thought about what he had said that last evening. It gave me a different perspective, and I saw his struggle in a new light. I realized the story about Jack wasn't really about money. It was about balance. He'd struggled to find balance between the challenges of career and family—one of the great struggles of the human condition. When things had become difficult, he'd buried himself in his work. It was the one thing he'd felt he could control.

When he needed to communicate, to resolve his indifferences, he had instead retreated into his comfort zone. Marcel Proust said, "We are healed of suffering only by expressing it to the full."

Talk to one another. Express it to the full.

The Things We Take for Granted

Do not dwell in the past, do not dream of the future,
concentrate the mind on the present moment.

—BUDDHA

*For each night of call, as interns in medical residency in 1997,
we go through all the cases the following morning with an attending physician. It is a time to learn, to ask questions, and to
defend our actions of the night before. We have not slept for
twenty-four hours. Physically we are exhausted; emotionally we
are numb.*

*Last night, a baby died upon delivery. We are nervous en-
tering the room. Dr. Hugh Randall Jr. walks to the front and
sits in the center. He is clearly aware of the previous night's
events. His face is blank, and his mood is less than cheerful. He
is a man of great wisdom and has little tolerance for medioc-
rity. We all envy his knowledge. He knows more about deliver-
ing a baby than almost anyone on earth. He spends his life at
the inner-city Grady Memorial Hospital, and delivers more
babies in a day than most physicians do in a week.*

He studies the fetal heart rate monitor strip and gets the history of the case. He turns to the chief resident. "What would you have done differently?" he asks.

"I would have taken her back for a C-section earlier."

He turns to another resident. "And you?"

"I would have used forceps."

He looks at the resident who actually delivered the baby. "Knowing what you know now, what would you have done differently?"

"Sir, the cord was wrapped so tightly around the baby's neck. There were no signs of distress until the very end. We tried to release it but couldn't reach it . . . I don't know what we could have done to make a difference."

Dr. Randall carefully looks back at the heart rate strip of the baby. He carefully studies the time line of events and the first signs of fetal distress. The quietness of the room makes us all feel uncomfortable. It seems like an eternity. We wiggle in our seats. I look at him and know that he feels entirely comfortable. He could have stayed in that moment for eternity.

He nods at the resident sitting in the hot seat. "I agree."

He puts down the chart and the heart rate strip. He pulls up a chair and directly faces the small crowd of people in front of him. The supreme court of our world has ruled.

"Sometimes there will be bad outcomes no matter what you do—even though you know you did everything you could." He looks around the room. "Is there anybody in this room who has never had a bad outcome?"

A few proud hands raise and wave like flags on a windy day.

"Well, if you're raising your hand right now, then you haven't delivered enough babies. Your time will come too. And it's probably closer than you think."

Spring of 2000

Fourth Year of Medical Residency

A T FIRST GLANCE, THE PHYSICAL THERAPY CENTER DIDN'T seem particularly special. It smelled of salty sweat. There was the expected equipment: the long parallel oak walking bars against a floor-to-ceiling mirror, an exercise bike, blue vinyl mats to stretch and roll around on, a small set of stairs to learn to climb again, and some scattered iron free-weights. But inside this small room, miracles happened—people regained their lives and their independence.

Matthew stood between the parallel bars—he was learning to walk again. He started down the long path in front of him. He was in his mid-fifties—tall with gray wavy hair and long slender arms. He wore blue cotton exercise shorts with white socks pulled up above his knees. He gripped the bars tightly—his knuckles white, arms trembling, and face grimacing. Each step for him was like running a mile. His legs felt like lead weights attached to his body. Sweat beaded up on his forehead and rolled down his temples.

Behind him stood a physical therapist. She was in her late twenties. She was petite but muscular and defined. She had one hand on a belt around his waist and one hand on his chest.

"All right, now, stand up straight," she said. She pushed her hand into his chest. "Look forward, not down … that's it … that's it."

Matthew tried to swing his hip forward and lift his leg without catching his toe.

"Good," the therapist said. "A little straighter, please." She pushed her hand into his lower back.

I stood at the doorway, with my shoulder resting against its frame, and smiled—I had just watched Matthew take his first steps on the road to recovering from an incomplete spinal cord injury.

Recently, Matthew had been involved in a motorcycle accident. He had bought the motorcycle on a whim. He'd recently sold a company that he had built from scratch. The profits had allowed him to live a life without having to worry about money. He had always dreamed of riding cross-country, the wind blowing through his hair; camping at Yellowstone; mountain biking in Colorado; hiking down the Grand Canyon.

Less than a week before leaving for a cross-country adventure, he'd gone to the store to get a carton of milk. As his motorcycle had turned left through the intersection, a car ran a red light and slammed into his back wheel. It sent him toppling through the air. He had landed on his back in the middle of the street. His legs wouldn't move. He'd fractured a bone in his back that had pushed into the spinal canal and injured his spinal cord. He'd undergone surgery to remove the pressure on his spinal cord, but the impairment remained. He was now learning to walk again through rehabilitation.

I walked up to him. "Do you mind if I cut in?" I asked the therapist.

"Did you see him walk?" she said as she smiled.

"I did," I said, also smiling.

I reached one hand around his belt and put my other hand forward against his chest. I said to Matthew, "Look at you—I'm so proud of you. You've come so far."

He leaned forward and turned his head toward me.

"Thank you," he said. "I tell you what amazes me—I used to define my life by how big of a deal I could take on and accomplish. How much money I could make. Do you know what defines success to me now?"

He stared down to the end of the parallel bars and nodded in that direction. "Making it to the end . . . when I can walk to the end. That is my new definition of success."

He grabbed the bars even harder, took a deep breath, and continued on.

∾

THE DAY BEFORE MATTHEW LEFT THE REHABILITATION HOSPI-tal, he handed me a small painting. "I wanted to show this to you," he said.

I held the painting in my hands and looked it over. It was a painting of a fisherman in the middle of a river. It was sunrise. Just enough light to make out the surroundings—to see the orange tint on the water, the mountains in the background.

The fisherman stood with his back toward the viewer, with his arms casting the line far into the distance. The fisherman could be anyone.

"It's a self-portrait," he said.

"A self-portrait?"

He smiled. "I began to take some art classes a few years back. My art teacher said the same thing. I guess he expected me to paint a picture of myself in a suit, with a dark background and a serious look on my face—perhaps the way that most businessmen want to be remembered. But that was never me . . . "

I handed the picture back to him, and he looked it over again.

"To me life was about freedom. I desired freedom to explore the world, to do the things that I wanted to do. Money was only a means to an end. It was never more than that. So when people talk about my success, I think they have a far different perception of success than I do."

I shared with him a story about asking my high school teacher why most artists were required to do self-portraits. "My teacher said that artists learn so much in painting a self-portrait because they are forced to look at themselves differently. They step outside themselves, and sometimes they see a different person. They often see something within themselves they never saw before."

He looked back down at the paining. "Your teacher was right."

Running Uphill

Aging is an issue of mind over matter.
If you don't mind, it doesn't matter.

—MARK TWAIN

It's Christmastime in New York City in 2007, and I walk down the city streets and take in the beauty of the holiday season. I walk past the illuminated snowflakes on the walls of Saks Fifth Avenue, the sparkling tree at Rockefeller Center, ice skaters in Central Park, and the elaborate window displays on Madison and Fifth Avenues.

I sit in a small bistro and look out the window. The streets are lined with people wrapped in long, dark overcoats and colorful scarves. After arriving at the dinner table, I struggle with reading the menu. I tilt a candle to try to illuminate it. No luck.

"The light is terrible in this place," I say.

My wife turns toward me and says in a concerned voice, "No... actually it's not."

I look at the couple across the table from us, some dear friends that came with us on the trip. "It's the letters, then. They're so small," I say.

They glance toward me and then at one another. "Not really, Scott," Trey says.

"Would you mind ordering for me?" I ask. I hand the menu to my wife. I feel helpless.

"I'll set up an appointment with the ophthalmologist next week," my wife says. I nod but don't say a word.

The ophthalmologist confirms what I have feared. I need reading glasses. My eyes are structurally sound, but the aging process has begun. There is no cure.

That night I sit in front of the mirror and notice the wrinkles across my forehead and the splintering lines beside my eyes. And for the first time in my life, I am confronted with the fact that I'm aging.

Summer of 2000

Fourth Year of Medical Residency

THE ROOTS OF PATRICK'S FAMILY TREE WERE DEEPLY entrenched in a small seaside town on the east coast of Ireland. Patrick claimed he was fifty-five, but he looked much older. Then again, his personality supported a younger age, so I never knew quite what to believe. His pale and freckled skin was deeply wrinkled from spending his youth in the sun. His glasses were so thick, his eyes seemed to jump out behind them.

He loved the Catholic church but was also fond of Guinness beer, dirty jokes, and beautiful women. He sprinkled his vernacular with profanity used in such good context that it didn't seem like profanity. He kept us all on our toes.

He was recovering from a total knee replacement for arthritis. It had begun with a limp and with his friends asking, "What's wrong? Why are you limping?" He'd gotten tired of the pain and the questions. He went to see an orthopedic surgeon. The X-ray had shown there was no space in his knee. "Bone on bone" is what the surgeon had told him.

"I don't know how you've been walking on this," the surgeon said.

"Ever tried hopping along on one leg? Try it; it's harder than it looks. So I just did my best to use both. Until I couldn't anymore," Patrick had said.

He was in rehabilitation trying to regain the range of motion of his knee. I walked into his room.

"Good morning, Patrick. How's that knee of yours?"

"Doing all right, I guess."

On his knee was a machine called a CPM. He called it a "torture device." The machine resembled a large knee brace that forced him to bend and extend his knee to regain the range of motion.

Each time his knee flexed and extended, his face grimaced as if he were exercising with too much weight.

"Is it too much?" I asked.

"No, it's fine."

"This whole aging thing is overrated, isn't it?" I said.

He laughed. "I wouldn't go back to my twenties for anything."

"Really? Are you serious?" I was again having trouble telling if he was joking.

"I'm very serious," he said. "Everybody my age complains of how this hurts and that hurts and how they wish they were younger, but they forget what it's like growing up. Don't get me wrong—I miss the good looks," he said with a laugh. "But I appreciate the wisdom."

I sat down beside him.

"I remember in grade school I used to have a bully that beat me up at the school yard a couple days a week. I lived in fear. He would steal my lunch money. He would take my head and bang it into things."

"You still remember that?" I asked.

"Absolutely—like it was yesterday. It still hurts. If I saw him today, sitting over there across this room"—he pointed to the corner—"I'd grab my cane and hobble over there and beat his arse with it," he said.

I laughed. His face remained serious.

"I also remember how tough it was to be a teenager. I had lots of pimples, and the kids used to tease me. I was insecure—a loner. It wasn't a fine time in my life. I look back now and realize that I was well into my forties before I felt comfortable in this world. Since then, my life has only gotten better."

"What got better?" I asked.

"Well, I settled down and got married. We had a few children, and life became very hard. In a way I lost myself, and I don't know exactly why. For some reason, I hit rock bottom emotionally. It took years to sort it out. I started to worry less, and I began to feel comfortable in my own skin. I was less concerned about what others thought," he said.

The machine was finished, his forced exercise for the day over.

His therapist walked into the room, a young beautiful girl with silky brunette hair and bronzed skin.

She smiled at him. "Are you ready for therapy?" she asked.

"Absolutely," he said. "Dr. Kelly, would you mind handing me my cane?"

I walked over and handed it to him. I helped him out of bed, and he put his arms on my shoulders and stood upright. He looked me in the eyes. He nodded toward the therapist across the bed. She was busy writing on his chart and not paying attention to us.

He then leaned up to my left ear and whispered, "And just because I'm a little older, doesn't mean I'm not young at heart— I still appreciate beautiful women."

She looked over at us and knew he was up to something. "All right, boys," she said.

He laughed.

He leaned his cane up against the wall and stood without assistance. He brought both hands toward his head and tapped his temples lightly with his index fingers. "Part of aging is what you make of it. A large part of it is up to you—it's in here."

He reached back for his cane and took a step. He was hunched forward and limped as he tried to walk. It seemed painful. I looked at his face, expecting to see him grimacing, but he was smiling instead.

∾

AT THE TIME I MET PATRICK, THE THOUGHTS OF AGING SEEMED so distant in my mind. Something that loomed in the horizon but never felt real. I felt immune, even though I saw it happen to everyone around me. Then aging struck me.

Since that day in New York, it seems that the process of aging has gained momentum. And yet, I have little fear. I find myself looking for ways to improve my physical presence through exercise and nutrition, but I also realize the importance of the spiritual and mental aspects of aging. Patrick opened that door for me. I am constantly trying to shift my focus to the present moment, without regrets and without trying to anticipate the future. It remains the one thing I can control.

I find myself in a very secure time in my life. The insecurities of growing up have long gone.

"Accept who you are," Patrick once said to me. Then he whispered, "But the real trick is, don't ever stop trying to improve."

I will continue trying until I take my last breath.

The Greatest Tool
in Medicine

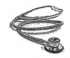

The first duty of love is to listen.

—Paul Tillich

Seven thirty in the morning in the summer of 1997—we wait impatiently to meet our attending physician in the hospital cafeteria. We are tired from a long night on call. He finally arrives. He is in his mid-sixties, with rounded shoulders, a silver full beard, and a determined look on his face. It is clear something is weighing heavily on his mind.

He sits down at the round table and pulls up a blue plastic chair. He places his coffee cup on the table. "Before we get started, I need to take a poll," he says. "What is the most important tool you have in medicine?"

We think about the newest tools and the latest gadgets at our fingertips.

"MRI," one resident says.

"Bypass grafts," yells another.

"Have you seen the new ultrasound machine for babies? It is unbelievable," a young resident chimes in.

The attending physician slowly shakes his head from side to side. A disappointed look spreads across his face. "No, your ears are," he says. He puts his index fingers behind each of his ears and pushes them out to the side so we can all see. "Your ears are your most important tool. Listen to your patients, young doctors, and they will tell you what is wrong with them."

Fall of 2000

Private Practice

AS KATIE READ THE NEWSPAPER ON AN EARLY AUGUST MORNing, she watched as the words danced across the page. But the words found their rightful place, and Katie went about her day. On her morning run, she felt a numbness burn through her thigh. It was sudden and intense and stopped her in her tracks. The sensation resolved and she continued running.

Maybe I'm just pushing myself too hard, she thought.

By her own admission, Katie was an overachiever. She had graduated at the top of both her college and business school, she trained for marathons, she was a faithful wife and a loving mother of two young children. She was now in her early thirties, and each challenge that came her way she took in stride.

A week later she felt transient numbness in her right hand. She thought, I need to slow down. I've got to slow down.

It went away as well.

She visited her primary care physician. He examined her and drew some blood. "You're right; you're pushing yourself too hard. You need to slow down. You have young children, you're trying to be a good wife, your career is demanding, and you're training for a marathon. Katie, you can't be everything to everyone. Go home; rest."

After leaving his office, she felt better. But the symptoms became more intense. The numbness began to involve her face. She felt as if she were having a stroke.

She visited her primary care physician again and was referred to a psychiatrist. He talked to her about the effects of stress on her body. "It might be causing some depression as well." He scribbled on a prescription pad. "Here, take this. This will help calm your nerves. And slow down," he said.

She rested. She stopped running, but the symptoms persisted.

She eventually ended up in my office. A friend had encouraged her to see me for another opinion. I sat and listened to her story.

"I know that these sensations are real, and I'm not crazy. Even if no one can find anything wrong. I just don't know where to turn. I've been scouring the Internet. The only thing I can come up with is multiple sclerosis. It says I need an MRI of the brain. Would you please order this for me?" she asked.

"Yes," I said. "I will."

"Really?" She looked at me with a relieved expression.

"Absolutely," I said. "I want to see you immediately after it's done, all right?"

"Thank you," she said. A wave of relief spread across her face.

The next afternoon my assistant handed me a piece of paper with a telephone number on it. "The radiologist is awaiting your call—she needs to speak with you about Katie," she said.

I dialed the phone number, knowing the news would not be good. It never is when the radiologist calls personally instead of sending you the report.

"I'm looking at this MRI of your patient," the radiologist said. "Tell me her clinical history."

I told her about Katie—a young woman with intermittent numbness and tingling and some occasional blurriness of vision. About a woman training for a marathon, and how she was pushing herself too hard, but in her heart knew something was wrong—and how I believed her.

"Well, she has multiple demyelinating lesions throughout her brain extending into her spinal cord. It looks like multiple sclerosis."

Katie had been right.

"I'm surprised she's doing as well as she is. I can't believe she's running," she said.

"I'm not. You would have to meet her to understand," I said.

I hung up the phone and turned toward my assistant. "Would you call Katie and tell her to come into the office today?" My assistant could see in my eyes that something was wrong.

I continued to see patients and tried to remain focused, but my mind continued to wander. I thought of the impact the disease would have on her life, her marriage, and her children. I tried to keep my mind clear.

An hour later, she sat back in the same examining room she'd been in the day before.

"What is it?" she asked. "Tell me."

I sat beside her and placed my hand on hers. "Katie, you were right all along. All the symptoms you felt were real. Not only that, you diagnosed yourself. It is multiple sclerosis."

"I knew it," she said.

She was laughing and crying at the same time.

She held a tissue in her hand and balled it up tightly. She patted the corners of her eyes. A faint smile remained on her face.

"I know that this is terrible news, but I'm relieved in a way to know that I'm not crazy—that what I was feeling was real," she said.

I knew exactly how she felt. For some patients the reaction to bad news is not what they'd expect. They feel a sense of relief. As if the weight of the world is lifted off of their shoulders. At least they know why they feel the way they do. Often they are reassured by a diagnosis—in their heart they already knew there was a problem.

Now Katie is being treated for multiple sclerosis in the hands of a wonderful neurologist. She has occasional exacerbations but is back to running. Even though her vision is occasionally blurry, she sees the world through a different set of eyes. And her vision of the world and of her life have never been clearer.

∾

I HESITATED TO INCLUDE THE STORY OF KATIE. THERE ARE FEW things I detest more than a doctor gloating on making a diagnosis that other physicians missed. This was not my intention. Her disease had progressed much more since the other doctors had evaluated her. Besides, I didn't make the diagnosis; Katie did. All I did was listen to her. She had told me what to do.

When a patient's symptoms fall outside the norm, I often think of Katie. She serves as a constant reminder to me to listen to my patients. She has made me a better physician. Her lesson has influenced other areas of my life as well. By listening, I have become a better father, husband, and friend.

And it remains true—regardless of the latest technologies we actively seek as physicians to improve quality of life and relieve pain—that the most important tools physicians will ever have are our ears.

Accepting Responsibility

Nothing strengthens the judgment
and quickens the conscience
like individual responsibility.

—Elizabeth Cady Stanton

It's the fall of 1993, and I am in my second year of medical school. A plastic surgeon is lecturing to us about a recent mission trip he took to South America. His is tall and athletic and wears a long white coat over blue scrubs. His demeanor is humble and gentle, but I can sense an underlying aura of confidence. As if he has found his purpose in life, and is not ashamed to admit he is good at what he does. He flips through slides on a carousel with the remote control in his hand.

Click.

"This young boy's cleft lip was so bad that he couldn't eat effectively. He was losing weight, and was ashamed to be seen in public," he said.

Click.

"*This is him after I fixed him.*" *The boy is smiling, with black hair that is neatly parted to one side. A thin line replaces the once large gap in his lip.*

Click.

"*This next young girl was born without an ear.*"

Click.

"*This is her after we made one for her.*" *The students look around the room at each other in amazement. It looks perfect.*

Click.

He goes through case after case, and each one is more impressive than the one before.

"*And the last slide I want to show you is not of the mission trip but a picture of a neighbor washing his car.*" *A man stands over a new red sports car and is washing it with his hands. A cigarette dangles out of his mouth.*

"*What's wrong here?*" *he asks.*

The crowd mumbles, but no one gives a definitive answer.

"*He's smoking . . . but cleaning his car by hand. Don't you see? He cares more about the car than he does about himself. That always struck me as odd. How do you love a car more than yourself?*

"*Serve others, young doctors. But, always remember—love yourself. Lights, please.*"

Late Fall of 2000

Private Practice

GEORGE WAS OBESE AND A DIABETIC. HE SMELLED OF SMOKE and alcohol, and his hands were stained with nicotine. The haze of the past night's drinking still loomed in his eyes. Cigarettes sat rolled up in his sleeve just above a faded Navy tattoo. He was now in his late fifties with a short crew cut. His demeanor was void of emotion.

George came in to see me on a Thursday afternoon because his hands and feet were becoming numb.

"It's annoying," he said. "I want it fixed." He then began a tirade about every doctor he had seen before me.

There was the vascular surgeon he was suing because the doctor couldn't save his big toe. A diabetic ulcer on his toe had turned into gangrene. By the time George showed up to the hospital it was too late. He was furious at his primary care physician for telling him that he was beginning to show signs of liver failure. George had a long history of drinking alcohol. In the mornings when he woke up, he snuffed out the hangover with a handful of Tylenol and a beer.

"Had he told me, I wouldn't have gotten drunk so much," he said.

Now it was my turn to treat George. His years of not eating properly and not taking his insulin as prescribed had taken a

toll on his nerves. I suspected George had developed a condition called peripheral neuropathy. I performed a test of his
nerves, and the responses were slow. It confirmed my suspi-
cions. I told him the results.

"I want it fixed," he said.

"George, there is no cure for this," I said. "We can give you
medication to treat the symptoms and improve your function, but you are going to have to help us in controlling your
diabetes."

"Of course there's a cure. And I don't want no pill that's going to cover it up and not fix it, either." He became agitated. "If
you have to cut me, then cut me. But I want it fixed."

"George, we need to talk."

While my other patients waited patiently, I sat beside
George with a calm voice and explained to him that the years
of neglecting his body had taken their toll. That smoking was
bad for him, and so was drinking alcohol in excess and mixing
it with Tylenol. I also talked to him about the importance of
taking his insulin and following his diabetic diet. I told him
that he was the one person who could help himself above all
others. Without his help, we could do nothing for him. He was
slowly committing suicide.

I watched as the wheels in his mind turned. He didn't
talk—he just listened and nodded his head. The layers of ne-
glect and denial slowly dissolved before my eyes.

At the end he said, "Thank you for taking the time to explain it to me."

He agreed to see a dietician. He would follow up with his
endocrinologist. He said he would stop smoking.

After seeing George that day, I thought about the patient-physician relationship. One of the hardest things I do as a doctor is managing expectations. With new technologies come increased expectations—sometimes unrealistic expectations.

If you have a joint that is riddled with arthritis, we can replace it. If your heart is failing, we can take a heart from a kind organ donor you've never met, and save your life. The advances in medicine are astounding, but we still don't know everything about the human body and medicine yet. We still have some work to do.

Like all good relationships, the physician-patient relationship takes the trust and commitment of two individuals. We know smoking is bad. We know at times we need to lose weight. We don't need to pay a doctor to tell us these things.

Bernie Siegel is a retired surgeon, writer, and loving soul. He used to tell patients: "Love yourself; if you do, then you will quit smoking."

"Love yourself." And let's perform some miracles together.

∾

AFTER SEEING GEORGE, I RECALL FEELING HOPEFUL ABOUT HIS prospects. He understood that he could control a part of his life. He might not have embraced responsibility, but it was something he knew he needed to accept. In his heart he knew it was in his best interests.

Later, I realized I took away much more from the encounter than I had offered. I began to communicate better with my patients. Often physicians do a poor job of communicating even the simplest messages, such as: "This is what I can I do for you, and I believe it can help you. But I need for you to do the following." Above all, the physician-patient relationship is based on communication and trust. In this quick-fix and rushed world, we need to realize that the outcomes will always be better if we work together.

Reasonable expectations are important in all relationships. That applies to relationships not just between a doctor and a patient; it applies to the husband and wife struggling in their marriage, the strained parent-child relationship, and the friendship that is losing its momentum.

"Love yourself," and you will be better able to love others. The world around you will silently fall into place.

Determining Your Own Fate

It is certain that habit, in man, eventually becomes
second nature, compelling him to practice that to
which he has become accustomed, regardless of whether
such a thing be beneficial or injurious to him...
The force of habit will triumph even over reason.

—Luigi Cornaro

*I place an MRI against the view box. It is the winter of 2000. I
show my patient and her husband the disc herniation pressing
against a nerve in her lower back.*

*"This is why you have the back pain and leg pain, and why
your leg is weak," I say.*

"Can I run today?" she asks.

*"Run?" I ask. "I can't imagine that with the pain you're in
you would want to run."*

*She begins to cry and leans her head into her husband's
chest. I sense something else is going on—something of greater
concern to her.*

"What is it?"

"She's run every day for the past three years. And she wants to continue," her husband says.

"Every day for three years? That's an amazing amount of discipline," I say.

"No, not really. It's more of a lack of discipline," she says, sobbing. "People that can run three days a week have discipline. For me, I have to do it every day of my life. Or I won't do it at all."

Winter of 2001

Private Practice

"JEFF, IF YOU CONTINUE ON THE SAME PATH YOU'RE ON RIGHT now," I said, "you'll be dead at fifty." Jeff looked up at me, and the reality of my words settled in.

I pointed out his family history. "Your father passed away at forty-eight from a heart attack. Your grandmother died of a stroke at age fifty. Your grandfather—fifty-one—heart attack." I reviewed his labs. "Your liver enzymes and cholesterol are elevated. You're overweight. You smoke and drink too much."

As the words rolled off my tongue, I found myself surprised at the directness of my approach. It was out of character for me to be so blunt, but for some reason I felt it was necessary. Maybe it was the cigarettes in his front pocket I had noticed as he entered the doctor's office. Or his disheveled appearance: the untucked shirt, the bloodshot eyes, the kerosene breath. Or maybe just the bravado of his attitude as he talked about staying out late drinking with his friends. "Sorry, Doc, big night," he'd told me.

At the age of thirty-three, he led the life of a college student headed down the wrong path. When he left my office that day, I didn't expect him to return. I thought he'd found another doctor, and I understood why. I reasoned that I might have lost a patient but maybe saved a life.

A year later, I opened the examining room and could not believe the man that stood in front of me. The last time I'd seen him had been a year ago. My patient, Jeff, was now a different person.

Jeff had lost ninety pounds. His hair was neatly combed to the side. His clothes were neatly pressed. The cigarettes were gone. "I have to be honest with you. When I left your office that day, I was angry. I drove around for two hours in my car thinking about what you said. You could have let it go, you know?" He paused. "But thinking back, it was exactly what I needed to hear.

"I came in today to show you how well I've done—and to prove you wrong."

I admired his discipline—I was also trying to find balance in my life. When I had entered into the real world of medicine, my life had become centered on building a medical practice. I'd worked diligently for many years to be in this position. And now that I was in practice, the long hours took a toll on my personal habits.

I told patients to exercise; when I left work the gym was closed. I told patients to stop and smell the roses; I barely stopped to breathe. I told patients to eat well; I didn't.

The hypocrisy of my actions took a personal toll on the way I felt about myself. Like it or not, physicians are role models. I needed to practice what I was preaching. And I wasn't. So I asked him how he had done it. Now I was the one receiving the advice.

"Well, I first looked at everything that I had tried and failed. Every time I failed on a diet, it was a crash diet. I would lose a few pounds, but after a week I would gain it back. Every time I started a new diet I swung for the fences, but I never stuck with it. I realized diets don't work. Lifestyle changes do."

He was holding a running magazine and pointed to it.

"The same was true of exercise. I would start a program and would think I could go out and run six miles—I couldn't. I would be so sore the next day, my new exercise program was over." He laughed. "I put the running shoes in the back of the closet for the next three years.

"So, instead, I set a time frame. I heard it takes twenty-one days to build a habit. I decided to go well beyond that and aim for three months. I modified my eating patterns and began to exercise. I'm not good at moderation with tobacco or alcohol, so I decided to quit them both that day. At one month, I decided I would reevaluate.

"The first two weeks were tough—but since I had committed to a time frame rather than a weight-loss goal, I just kept going with it. At about week two, I started feeling better. I added a multivitamin each morning. I stopped drinking soft drinks and began drinking water. I cut out the bread, pastas, and the wheat. I began walking and then progressed to running."

I could see the enthusiasm in his face and hear it in his voice.

"Each week got a little better. By the first month, the smell of cigarettes made me cringe. The smell of smoke slowly faded from my clothes. It was nice to wake up without a hangover. The weight came off. By the end of the first month, I couldn't believe my eyes. I stepped on the scale one morning and realized I had lost twenty-five pounds. That was all the inspiration I needed. From then on I just continued to add positive habits into my life."

I thought about what he said and how it applied to my life. "So, just a change in habits—that's it?"

"Exactly—your habits will define who you are and what you become. I began to study about habits when I began seeing success. You become in life what you think about. Habits can be the difference between success and failure, strong or weak relationships, even life or death."

His voice softened. "I learned the hard way that a habit sneaks into your subconscious mind. We begin to perform actions without conscious thought. Before we realize it, it's become a patterned behavior. Patterned behaviors will ultimately define who you are as a person. Good habits can take you to a whole new level if you let them. Bad habits can kill you if left unchecked. The problem is the subconscious mind doesn't know the difference between a good habit or a bad habit. The trick is to rewire the subconscious mind to understand the difference," he said.

I could have talked to him for hours, but patients were waiting. I was mesmerized by his candor. Although many had tried and failed, he had realized success through consistency of action.

"I used to see myself as a fat person. Now I don't. I used to see myself as a smoker. Now I don't. I used to see myself as an alcoholic. Now I don't."

"That's the difference?" I asked.

"Yes."

He taught me that life shouldn't be about hitting the home run. It's more about stepping up to the plate and swinging. You might get a single or a double, and occasionally you'll strike out. But if you keep swinging, you'll find your way home.

∾

ABOVE MY DESK IN MY WRITER'S STUDIO, TYPED ON WHITE linen paper and thumbtacked to the wall, is a quote from Luigi Cornaro:

> It is certain that habit, in man, eventually becomes
> second nature, compelling him to practice that to
> which he has become accustomed, regardless of
> whether such a thing be beneficial or injurious to him.
> The force of habit will triumph even over reason.

Below it I added Jeff's words: "Your habits will define who you are and what you become. Habits can be the difference between success and failure, strong or weak relationships, even life or death."

Both of these quotes serve as a constant reminder that life is a matter of choices. I have the choice to choose my habits, so I must choose them wisely. And, for me, those simple words have made all of the difference.

What We Don't See

The more serious the illness, the more
important it is for you to fight back,
mobilizing all your resources: spiritual,
emotional, intellectual, physical.

—Norman Cousins

*We stand outside a patient's door in the outpatient clinic. It's late
in my third year of medical school in 1995. My senior year looms
just around the corner. My attending physician picks up the chart
from the door and glances over it. "It looks like this patient is here
with the chief complaint of fibromyalgia. Do you believe in fibromyalgia?" he asks me.*

*"I'm not sure. I believe there is something there, but there is
no test to confirm it," I say.*

*"I understand. I never believed in it either. Then one day my
wife began to complain of pain everywhere in her body. I couldn't
make sense of it. We went from specialist to specialist and couldn't
get a straight answer. All blood work was negative, and all imag-
ing studies showed nothing. A rheumatologist diagnosed her with*

fibromyalgia. At first, I was skeptical and thought he was trying to pacify us. I didn't want to be pacified. I asked him why no one had diagnosed her with this before. 'Probably because they didn't want to tell you the truth,' he said. 'But, that's what it is.'"

He glances down at the chart again and looks through it. "I see the way she struggles to get out of bed every morning, and the constant pain she lives with every day. And now I never question if it's real or not."

He tucks the chart under his arm, opens the patient's door, and walks in.

Spring of 2001

Private Practice

"THE HARDEST PART OF DEALING WITH CHRONIC PAIN IS that it has no boundaries. It affects every part of your life. It doesn't discriminate—nothing in your life is spared," Emily said.

On a Friday morning, Emily was stopped at a red light on her way to work. As she looked in the rearview mirror, she noticed a car approaching fast. She saw the driver wasn't paying attention. She gripped the steering wheel with all of her strength. He never put on his brakes.

The moment she was struck, she felt a pop in her back and pain down her leg. Her leg suddenly became weak. At the emergency room, they did an MRI and found she had fractured a bone and a nerve was being pinched. The pain was severe and constant.

A spine surgeon was called into the hospital. He told her that she needed surgery.

"Anything to get rid of this pain," she said. Off to the operating room they went.

The surgeon was meticulous and stabilized the fracture; he removed the pressure from the nerves. He re-approximated her skin with a plastic surgeon's stitch to minimize her scar. Her function returned, but her pain stayed.

"This doesn't make sense—everything went so well," he said. He repeated the MRI of her spine. "It should go away," he said. "The nerves are free of pressure, and the MRI looks good. Let's give it more time."

She did, but time didn't heal her. Eventually she ended up seeing a pain specialist. He tried injections of steroids around her nerve—the pain lessened but persisted. He tried medicine to calm her nerves—it didn't work. He put her on high doses of narcotics that took away the pain. The downside was that it impaired her judgment, and she didn't like the way it made her feel. Eventually, through the process of trial and error, a medication was found that helped her pain but didn't impair her cognition.

I saw her in the office on a Tuesday morning. I opened the back of her gown and looked at the incision. I reviewed her MRI and talked to her about how this event had changed her life.

"There is nothing in my life that this did not change," she said as she looked down at the ground. "My husband was supportive initially, but after years of hearing me complain, he left. And to tell you the truth, I understood. I didn't want to live with me either."

"And your children?" I asked.

"Well, they still live with me and are still trying to understand. But I know that they're tired of hearing it too." She began to cry, and I handed her a box of tissues. "At school last year, my five-year-old made a Christmas list for Santa, and all it said was for Mommy to not be in pain. No toys, no puzzles, nothing for her."

"How about your job?" I asked.

"Well, they fired me—I lost that also. I have disability, but it barely pays for the medication. And when I tell people I'm on disability, they look at me differently. They don't understand I want to work—I just can't."

I asked what she liked least about going to the doctor's office. "Asking for pain medication. I just wish the doctors understood that if it was up to me, I wouldn't be on anything."

I nod my head in agreement—a common complaint.

"You know, we really take our bodies for granted. They perform so well that we don't pay much attention to them until something goes wrong: a lump in our breast, our heart skipping a beat, a rash—for me it was pure and intense pain," she said.

Two days later I received a medical journal in the mail. The headline read, "Doctor goes to trial for prescribing patient narcotics." I read through the article, and it told how the government was threatening to revoke the doctor's license for prescribing pain medication to his cancer patients. Often, an investigation is warranted when a physician abuses his role. In this case it appeared that a well-respected physician was a target of a much bigger problem. The physician wasn't the first, but neither would he be the last.

I think about Emily and realize she's not alone. There are millions of Americans in chronic pain, and we have no great answers for them. Our tests often come up normal, and we try to offer explanations to ease their mind and let them know their pain is real. They deserve more than having their government and their physicians turn their backs on them.

∾

ONE BEAUTIFUL SPRING EVENING, I WENT OUT TO THE MAILBOX and spoke briefly to my neighbor across the street. She was in her mid-fifties, pleasant, and always wearing a smile. We talked for a few brief moments, then I went into my house to be with my family.

A week later, a neighbor asked me if I'd heard the news. "You know she passed away last week."

I thought about the last time I'd seen her. She had looked healthy and happy.

"Was it a car accident?"

"No, she died of a brain tumor. She was diagnosed six weeks ago."

When I heard this, I thought of Emily because she reminded me about how illness and pain carry over into other people's lives. My neighbor had seemed so cheerful, and yet she had carried a terrible burden.

When the door to the examining room is shut, people open their hearts to their physicians and tell them the truth about their lives. I am often humbled and find myself thinking, If I saw this person on the street, I never would have known the challenges they are facing. The mental aspects of their illness and the pain are carried with them regardless of where they go. They can't be seen or touched, but they're forever present. It serves as a reminder to me to give people the benefit of the doubt, because I never know what they're dealing with in the privacy of their homes. What consumes them behind closed doors?

Be gentle with one another. You never know what those around you are carrying in their minds and in their hearts.

Life Is Fragile

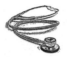

Life is no brief candle to me. It is a sort of
splendid torch, which I have got a hold
of for the moment. And I want to make it burn
as brightly as possible before handing it
on to future generations.

—George Bernard Shaw

I sit at the end of a long oak table in the summer of 1999. An attending surgeon lectures about unusual clinical presentations and the intricacies of determining the correct diagnosis. I have finished the workday, but the fatigue of a long night of being on call makes my eyelids heavy, and I long for a warm bed.

A resident next to me squirms and rolls his eyes. He whispers under his breath, "It's not like we're going to ever see any of this stuff. What a waste of time."

The attending hears his mumbling. "Do you have something to say to everyone?" he asks.

*"I'm sorry, but I've never seen any of this in clinical practice,"
the resident says.*

The attending walks beside the table and stops directly across from the resident. He rests his hands against the table and leans forward, looking the resident directly in the eye.

"Oh really? Well, always remember what I am about to tell you: Just because you haven't seen it, doesn't mean it hasn't seen you. And if you miss it—just once—you'll turn around and your patient will be dead." He snaps his fingers. "Like that."

We all look at one another and slowly sink into our seats. The gravity of the profession I have chosen settles in. Suddenly, I'm alert and wide awake.

Fall of 2001

Private Practice

I OPENED THE DOOR, WALKED INTO THE EXAMINING ROOM, and saw Nadine leaning against the examining table. As she saw me, she quickly stood and embraced me. Each time Nadine came to my office she hugged me and planted a kiss on either cheek. She was French, and that was her custom. Who was I to interfere? And so I obliged. Each time I saw her, she made my day better.

Nadine's hair was long and flowing and sprinkled with subtle grays. Though in her mid-fifties, her facial features defied the aging process. Her skin was void of lines and flawless.

"I began to have a sore throat about five days ago. I want to get it treated because I am leaving for France tomorrow to see my father," she said. America was where she'd resided for the past fifteen years, but her heart remained in her hometown— a small island off the coast of France.

I shone a light into her mouth. It was red and swollen. It looked angry. I swabbed the back of her throat with a Q-tip and sent a rapid strep test to the lab. I gently palpated her lymph nodes under her chin, just in front of her ears, and down her neck. As we talked I continued to examine her.

"Is he okay?" I asked.

"No, he is not doing so well. My father was diagnosed with colon cancer about four years ago."

She looked toward the ground and swung her crossed legs gently back and forth as if she was embarrassed to tell me something.

"He originally put his faith in Western medicine. He under- went surgery. He tried chemotherapy. But the side effects—the nausea, vomiting, dizziness—he eventually decided the quality of his life was more important than duration. He chose a natu- ral route: eating well, vitamins, exercise, strengthening the rela- tionships around him." She looked at me for approval.

"I understand—he's not alone," I said.

"It was hard at first to accept it. But our family tried to re- spect his decision. He fared well until just recently. My mother called and said it is time to say good-bye."

She told the story without tears, but a sadness was evident in her body language, her facial expression, and her glazed brown eyes.

"The one thing I am grateful for is we were granted the gift of time. We were able to say good-bye. Since the day he was diagnosed, my dad and I wrote letters to each other each week. We made up for lost time. We are closer now than ever. I have said good-bye little by little over the past four years."

As always, Nadine saw the dim ray of hope in the darkest of moments.

I checked the rapid strep test, and it was positive. I handed her a prescription for antibiotics.

"Give your father my best," I said.

"I will."

I thought of her occasionally, wondering how she was coping with her father's imminent death. We assume as physicians that when people don't come to see us, they're healthy and their life is busy. If they need us, they'll let us know.

I received some bad news on a Tuesday afternoon when the weather was changing and the first cool crisp of fall blew through the air. A friend of hers came to see me.

"How's Nadine?" I asked.

She looked at me with a concerned and puzzled expression. "You haven't heard?"

"No," I said. "I'm afraid I haven't."

"Doctor, Nadine was involved in a car accident in France. She and her husband had left after having dinner with their son. It was raining, and a car lost control and hit them. Her husband and her son lived... but Nadine died at the scene."

I had trouble finding words to speak.

"I thought you knew," she said. "I felt sure of it, or I would have told you earlier."

After she left, I went back to my office and closed the door. I felt like someone had punched me in the stomach—that deep, nauseating feeling that lingers long after you expect it to leave. I thought about how life can change in a moment, and how we often take people for granted—as if they will always be with us.

I wish I could see Nadine one more time, to give her a hug and a kiss on each cheek, and to tell her how much I miss her.

And to tell her good-bye.

❧

AT THE END OF EVERY HOT AND HUMID SUMMER, THE FIRST crisp wind of fall blows in. Sometimes it's late September, but often it patiently waits until mid-October. To me it has always marked a new beginning—a time for me to pause and look at my goals for the year ahead. Where do I want to go, and how do I want to get there?

After Nadine's death, the first fall breeze took on new meaning. It reminded me to take an afternoon off and to reflect. It prompted me to anchor my prayers around gratitude for all the many things that have blessed me: for my health, my family, my career, my friendships, my struggles, and my accomplishments. My goals for the year had to wait until later.

It reminded me to simply live in the present.

Losing a Loved One

Death leaves a heartache no one can heal,
love leaves a memory no one can steal.

—ON A HEADSTONE IN IRELAND

*I'm in sixth grade, in middle school. We look outside at the play-
ground, anxiously awaiting recess. We can see the sun beaming
through the rectangular window on the steel metal door. We feel
like we are in prison.*

*The middle school principal walks into our classroom in a
brown polyester suit. He stands in front of us with a determined
look on his face. There is a light chatter of young voices in the
background. His voice suddenly booms through the room.*

"Quiet please… I need your attention."

*The chatter stops quickly. We see his face is serious and his
mood somber.*

*"One of your classmates, Phillip… his father died yester-
day. I need to ask each of you to be extra kind. It is going to
be a rough year for him." When he leaves, we all say a prayer
for Phillip.*

I look at the seat next to me, Phillip's seat, and see that it's empty. And now I know why.

When Phillip returns to school, I make a special effort to go out of my way to be nice to him. He comes to my house often; we ride bikes and play together. But we never talk about his father. It's too painful for him. Well, at least, I know it would be too painful for me.

Looking back—I believe a part of me was bargaining with God. I thought if I were nice to Phillip, then maybe God would have mercy on me—and not take my father too.

Winter of 2002

Private Practice

MICHAEL GREW UP IN A SMALL, CROWDED APARTMENT IN Brooklyn, New York. The once red bricks had turned brown from the exhaust of Yellow Cabs and from the ash of fires burning throughout the winter to keep the city warm.

His father was an Italian immigrant who worked at a local butcher shop. It was the only trade he knew when he'd arrived from Italy, and as a third-generation butcher, he was an artist at carving beef. His mother cleaned apartments to buy the few extras: a Monopoly game, winter clothes from the Salvation Army, but most importantly an old record player for her husband, so he could sing along and enjoy Italian opera.

His voice was strong and bold—sometimes too powerful. Anchored by the voice of their father, the children would sing along. When he sang too loudly, the neighbor would bang his fist against the wall, and they would curl up under the blankets and laugh.

For Michael, his father was the man he admired most in the world and his best friend. If his father wasn't at work, he was with his son. They took long walks together each evening. They played catch with old worn gloves and a ratty baseball. His dad saved every penny he could to take his son to see the prizefights.

When Michael was twelve, his father went to the hospital with a cough and a fever. He never came home. And Michael was never the same.

His mother broke the news. Her eyes were red and glassy. "Your father . . . he passed away at the hospital. He was a good man. God must have needed him in heaven." She was deeply religious, and as she talked to Michael, she clutched a Bible with her right arm against her chest. Michael felt as though someone had reached into his chest and pulled out his heart.

At his wedding, an Italian friend sang his father's favorite song in his honor—"Ave Maria." His beautiful voice echoed throughout the church: "*Aaaaah veeeh maaa rrrrrheeeeee eee-aaaaaa.*"

Michael stood up at the front of the church, as tears rolled down both cheeks, and he bit his lip to control himself. Years of built-up emotion still lingered in him.

I met him in his early eighties. He had moved to Atlanta to be closer to his grandchildren. I saw him frequently and always enjoyed his company. Each time he came to see me, he would never forget to ask me one question: "How's the family?" It was sincere and honest—he meant it.

Over time, I opened up more and more. I told him about my close relationship with my father. I talked to him about my wife and my children.

"Never take your relationship with your father for granted," he said. "You just never know."

"Yeah, I try not to," I said. I told him about our Saturday morning golf games and our trip to Ireland. How supportive he is of me. How much I admire him.

Michael said, "I still think of my father often. When he passed, the whole foundation of my life was ripped beneath me. There was nothing below. My mom did her best, but it was tough. He was a good man—the person that meant the most to me in the world. I still wonder what it would be like to get to know him better. I still miss him."

"After all these years?"

"Absolutely."

His eyes welled up with tears, and he bit his lip. "Time may lessen the burden, but it never takes away the pain. You never get used to losing a parent. Nothing can fill that void."

ꙮ

AT THE TIME OF THIS WRITING, IT WAS JUST BEFORE DAYBREAK. The world was remarkably still. There was no wind, and silence filled the air. I sat down to think about my parents and what they have meant to me. Almost immediately I sank into a deeper and more loving place.

I have been very fortunate; both of my parents are alive and well. They have each lived a full life and had the pleasure of raising children and enjoyed the gift of grandchildren. They married over fifty years ago and have a thriving friendship and understand what the term "unconditional love" truly means. They have proven to me that it is possible to commit to someone for your entire life.

As a child, I thought that the most devastating thing that could happen to me would be to lose a parent. My parents were the foundation of my life. A part of that stability in my life remains because they are still here. I find great comfort in knowing I can pick up a telephone and hear the gentle voice of my father on the other end of the line. His voice alone has calmed me down in many situations long before I fully appreciated the wisdom of his words. A simple hug from my mother often turned a bad day into a good one.

Michael taught me to appreciate their presence, but more importantly their friendship. They were once the people that navigated the world for me, and now sometimes they lean on me too. It's something I take great pride in.

Being a physician has been a constant reminder that no one lives forever, and that I must confront the inevitable. I've had many years to prepare and to face what I know will eventually come. But in my heart, I know that no matter how hard I try, I will never be ready to let them go.

Beautiful Love

I believe that imagination is stronger than knowledge—
That myth is more potent than history.
I believe that dreams are more powerful than facts—
That hope always triumphs over experience—
That laughter is the only cure for grief.
And I believe that love is stronger than death.

—Robert Fulghum

It was my fourth year of medical residency in the late spring of 2000. Across the front of Caroline's chart were the words: "Do Not Resuscitate" written in black marker. She and her husband had decided against prolonging the inventible. Her lungs were failing her, and even the simple act of breathing was a struggle. So when she took her last breath, the nurses and I didn't say a word. We placed a white sheet over her head and waited for her husband to return.

Her husband, Peter, had been by her side since the day she was admitted. Each night he slept beside her in a reclining chair. He would comb her hair and rub her feet with lotion. When she cried, he would hold her and sing to her in a quiet voice. She died while he went to get a cup of coffee. It didn't surprise me. Some things in life don't need an explanation.

I stood outside her room and thought of how to break the painful news to Peter that his wife had died and he was now left to face the world alone. I was no further along from the moment I started when I saw him walk down the hall toward me.

When he approached me he said, "She's gone, isn't she?"

I nodded. As his knees began to buckle, I reached out and eased him into a chair outside her room. He held his head in his hands and cried. "I need to see her," he said. "Can I?"

I stood outside the door to make sure his last moments with his wife were without interruption. I saw him pull the sheet from over her head. He lifted her lifeless hand and sat beside her and talked to her. When he was done, he leaned over and kissed her on the forehead. He replaced the white sheet over her head and walked toward me.

"Thank you," he said. He put my hand in his and placed his other hand on top. "Thank you for everything." He walked out down the same hall he'd entered. The elevator door closed, and I never saw him again.

That night at dinner, my wife and I were seated next to a table where two middle-aged women sat. With each glass of wine they drank, their voices resonated more loudly throughout the restaurant.

"Are you all right?" my wife asked.

I nodded.

"Anything to do with me?" she asked.

"No."

"*There are no good men in the world anymore,*" the woman next to me said. "*Not a damn one.*" The women raised their glasses, toasted each other, and laughed.

Not true, I thought. I met a great man today. His name is Peter.

Spring of 2002

Private Practice

WILLIAM AND ELIZABETH SPENT THE LAST FIFTY-NINE years of their marriage walking through life holding hands together. They were now in their mid-eighties. William was slightly taller than Elizabeth, and he used a cane for walking. Elizabeth needed a cane but didn't use one for the sake of vanity. Each time I saw them, they wore the same outfits—just different colors. He wore a wool cap and a wool blazer, even in the humidity of the hot Atlanta sun. She wore a skirt but was more in tune with the changes of weather. In the summer it was light cotton, and in the winter a heavy wool—but always a skirt.

Over the years their gait had adapted to their changing needs. It had once been more upright and brisk but had now evolved to be more slow and cautious. The risk of losing their balance and falling was a reality. As one began to lose balance, the other offered an arm in support. They looked out for each other.

Their cautious eyes scanned the sidewalks, to look for potential areas of trouble: uneven pavement, a drop-off, or a hole. Their spines had become slightly bent forward over the years, allowing them to see what lay ahead and the danger below.

On a clear spring morning, William and Elizabeth walked into my office with a difference of opinion and wanted me to be the judge.

"Dr. Kelly, please tell Elizabeth she has to wear pants. We can't keep having her bump into things and get these horrible cuts on her leg," William said.

I surveyed the wound, and William was right. Her fragile skin was as thin as rice paper—if I held it to the light, the beam would shine right through. Her skin tore each time she bumped into an object, and stitches wouldn't hold her wounds together. So we would re-approximate the skin with little strips of sterile tape and apply antibiotic ointment and wrap it up. And I would tell her to be more careful.

A month later, she walked in holding William's hand, with blood trickling down her leg. William was beside himself. She smiled with a broad grin.

I had slapped her on the wrist too many times, I thought.

"Elizabeth, you have to wear pants. Each time you come in here the cuts get worse. William is just trying to look out for you. I'm going to have to side with him this time."

She looked at me, disappointed. "But I've worn skirts for the last eighty years and I've never liked pants. I'll try, but I can't promise anything." She and William then stood up, and they reached out for each other. They interlocked fingers and walked out together.

Two weeks later she was back with a cut on the opposite leg.

"Doctor, I tried to tell her what you said. I told her—I did. But she just refuses to wear pants," William said.

She looked at me and winked. That was the moment I understood she was never going to wear pants. Each time I fixed her wounds, we talked, and our friendship grew.

I learned how their families had lost everything in the Great Depression. How it felt to be broke and scared. They revealed there had been a time in their marriage when they had almost separated. Apparently, another woman had been trying to gain William's attention and he'd been tempted—and Elizabeth had found out and became furious and jealous. She'd put a stop to it. In the end, it had strengthened their marriage.

I learned how hard it was to lose a child in a car accident, and the deep hurt of burying a child. I learned about their travels, their passion for dancing, and how he regretted fighting in a war. He loved his country, but he loved his wife more.

I received a call on a Monday morning from William and Elizabeth's daughter.

"I'm so sorry to bother you. But last week my mother, Elizabeth, died."

"I'm so sorry," I told her.

"Unfortunately, it gets worse. My father, William, died about four days later. It's been a rough week." Her voice quivered. "They thought the world of you, and I thought you would want to know."

"What happened?"

"We don't really know. She died in her sleep. But, of course, he didn't do well—you know how close they were. He cried day and night. When we came to check on him one morning, he had passed also."

I sensed her loss with each word she spoke. How hard it must have been to lose one parent, much less both within a week.

"The doctor asked me if I wanted an autopsy on him. He said it was very unusual he died so suddenly. I'm just a little confused, and I didn't know where to turn. You knew them so well. What do you think I should do?"

"What do you think he died from?" I asked.

"I don't know. It sounds silly, but I think he died of a broken heart. Do you think something like that is possible?" she asked.

I leaned back in my chair and thought about the last time I had seen them together: how William had stroked Elizabeth's hair when I cleaned her wounds, the way he had looked at her when he talked to her, and how he'd held her cheeks when he kissed her.

"Yes," I said. "It's possible. I think he died of a broken heart. I don't think an autopsy is necessary."

"Me either." I could hear the peace in her voice.

When we hung up the phone, I closed the door to my office and thought about my wife. I understood why William didn't want to live without her, and how he couldn't bear to face the world alone.

I just hope and pray that if I am ever in a similar situation, someone will stand up for me. No autopsy necessary. I would ask that the extra effort be diverted to the following cause. I would rather my death certificate read exactly as follows: "Cause of death—broken heart (he missed his wife)."

And then I will rest in peace for eternity.

∾

THREE MONTHS AFTER MY LAST OFFICE VISIT WITH WILLIAM and Elizabeth, I received an invitation to their sixtieth anniversary party. It was intended to be a small gathering of family, but they insisted that I be included on the guest list. I was honored, but out of respect for the intimacy of a family gathering and due to the business of starting a new practice, I declined. To this day, it remains on my long list of regrets. While trying to keep my head above water, I'd missed their last anniversary here in this life together.

A few weeks later they stopped by the office. They filled me in on the details—the singing and dancing and laughter and tears. They made me promise I would be at the next one. They walked out of my office that day holding hands and left me with a smile. They taught me that love can endure. I still find great comfort in the hope.

Do I still believe that it's possible to die of a broken heart? You bet I do. I always will.

Conclusion

I OFTEN THINK BACK TO THE FATEFUL DAY IN THE FALL OF 1994, in my third year of medical school, when I wrote in my journal for the first time. I envision a younger version of myself sitting alone in my office with hardwood floors and books and notes scattered across my desk. I see a young man struggling to find his place on this earth. I recall his pure intentions and dreams of saving the world, but I sense the sadness in his heart. I want to go back and talk to him, to sit beside him and share with him what I've learned. I want to lessen his pain.

What would I say?

Love yourself. Always choose a path that inspires you. Watch the sunrise. Pray not for what you want but be grateful for the abundance in your life. Meditate. Travel. Don't take life for granted. Listen. Serve others. Forgive. Take care of yourself. When you find the one, reach out, hold her hand, and never let go. Slow down. Look forward to being a father, as it is more rewarding than you ever imagined. Accept the bad with the good—sometimes you need to feel a little pain to awaken you to the good in your life. Make time to be alone and reflect; it will make you a better husband, father, and friend. Live your life in the present. Let go of the past and stop trying to control the future. And don't forget to cherish those you know and love. Don't take them for granted. But also remember: In the mines of humanity there are many undiscovered gems. Open your heart to others even though it might get hurt—it will heal.

Look across the street. There's a young boy playing catch with a red rubber ball. I can see him. Push your textbooks and notes aside, walk across the street, and play catch with him. Toss the ball into the air. Don't hold back. Watch him smile, and don't forget to smile and laugh with him.

Reach out to your patients sooner rather than later. Listen and take good notes. Open your heart and trust in them. They will show you the way.

How do I know for sure?

My patients taught me so.

Acknowledgments

FOR MY WIFE, DEBORAH—THE STRONGEST WOMAN I KNOW. Thank you for your support and love. Life's journey wouldn't be the same without you.

To my girls, Caelyn and Elizabeth. When you entered this world, a new life began for me. My heart belongs to you.

To my parents, Don and Terre Kelly. You are the cornerstones of my life and prove that unconditional love is possible.

For my brother and sister, Mark and Lisa. When I think of growing up together, all I remember is love.

For my dear friend and father-in-law, Sonny Bonner—a man of character and unwavering faith. You lived your life placing the needs of your family above your own. All men would do well to follow in your footsteps. And for Barbara Bonner, you exemplify what a mother-in-law, wife, and friend should be.

For Warner, my other brother. Kindred spirits belong together. Art heals.

For Natalie, Tyler, Matthew, and Michael. When I married the woman of my dreams, I didn't know I would be so blessed to have all of you enter my life.

I would like to thank my editor, Paul McCarthy, for his unstinting support and for wielding my words into prose that I look upon with great fondness. Big hugs.

For Susanne Lakin and Anne Newgarden, for polishing the manuscript into its final form. For Karen Minster, for the beautiful design of the interior of the book and her patience and support. Many thanks to Laura Duffy for her artistic vision of the cover. For Kem Lee, a wonderful photographer and true artist.

I want to thank my patients for trusting in me and sharing their wisdom. It has been a privilege and an honor caring for you. You have helped me grow into the man that I am today. And for that, I am eternally grateful.